I0157338

KICKSTART YOUR RECOVERY - THE ROAD LESS TRAVELED TO FREEDOM FROM ADDICTION

BY TAITE ADAMS

Kickstart Your Recovery

Rapid   Response   Press
1730 Lighthouse Terr., Suite 12
So   Pasadena,   FL   33707
www.rapidresponsepress.com
Ordering   Information:
Quantity sales. Special discounts are available on quantity purchases by corporations, associations, and others. For details, contact the publisher   at   the   address   above.
Orders by U.S. trade bookstores and wholesalers. Please contact Rapid Response Press: Tel: (866) 983-3025; Fax: (855) 877-4736 or visit www. rapidresponsepress.com.
Printed in the United States of America

Publisher's   Cataloging-in-Publication   data
Adams,   Taite.
A title of a book : a subtitle of the same book / Taite Adams.
p.   cm.
ISBN   978-0-9889875-0-0
1. The main category of the book —Health —Other category. 2. Another subject category —Mind and Body. 3. More categories — Recovery.

Second Edition

==================

Limit of Liability/Disclaimer of Warranty

================

Disclaimer

================

Medical Disclaimer

To my son - Your light and growth provides a constant source of joy and pride;

To Mom - Who loved me even when I didn't;

To my love - There are times when I think I can't possibly love you more. And then I do. You are my best thing.

Get All The Books In The Series:

Opiate Addiction - The Painkiller Addiction Epidemic, Heroin Addiction and The Way Out

Safely Detox From Alcohol and Drugs at Home

Restart Your Recovery - 12 Things You Can Do To Get Back on the Beam

Who is Molly?: Molly Drug Facts, What is Ecstasy, and Life-Saving MDMA Effects Info

See http://www.TaiteAdams.com for more info

Contents

Kickstart Your Recovery

Preface

This book, or Guide, has been on my mind for quite some time. I looked for something along these lines when I started my journey many years ago and didn't find anything that answered my multitude of questions. I don't know that there can ever be one little book that can give solace to all of those doubts and fears, but maybe something that can help just a little bit would be a great start. I am not an expert or an authority on anything. What I am is someone who has been to the bottom and was granted relief and a new life. Was this difficult? Actually the difficult part was getting to "the end" - getting to that point where I had had enough and was ready to cry "uncle" and get some help. After that, it really wasn't so bad.

I do see people on a daily basis that fit along the entire spectrum, though, of being entirely ready to "do this", just not sure, or completely clueless as to what has them in a vice-like grip, if anything. This is what is so frustrating, sad and cunning about the disease of addiction. So many of us will fight it to the death, literally, while others will "give up" and recover - going on to lead beautiful, happy and useful lives. I have lived stages of my life all along this spectrum and, luckily, I was able to get to a point of desperation and surrender before this thing took everything or, worse yet, killed me or someone else. I became willing to get help and clung to everything that was offered to me. It worked and continues to work on a daily basis.

The control freak in most of us, at least those of you who would search out a book of this sort, still wants to know what is in store for them if they do decide to "do this" or even if already in early recovery. Perfectly understandable. There's only so much "letting go" a newcomer can do, after all. What I've catalogued here is essentially a Newcomer's Guide to Recovery. I've attempted to answer all of the questions that I hear in meetings and from newcomers, as well as many of the ones that I had in the beginning. I am an active member of Alcoholics Anonymous and, as such, very much respect their Traditions. Because of this, my real name was not used in the publishing of this book. However, every experience related herein was absolutely real and shared in the heartfelt hope that it touches at least one person and makes a difference in their journey to recovery.

How Did I Get Here?

It ain't what you don't know that gets you into trouble. It's what you know for sure that just ain't so.   -Mark Twain

Many of us could probably add the word "Again" to that question. Chances are, life isn't going according to plan at the moment or you would not have purchased and be reading this book. Trust me, I get it. One of the hardest things to come to terms with is the fact that there is something that may have an iron-clad grip on our lives and, no matter how hard we try to wriggle and scheme our way out, the noose just keeps getting tighter.   Do you think that you may have a problem with alcohol or drugs? Here's a hint: Most people that aren't alcoholics or addicts don't sit around wondering if they have a problem with alcohol or drugs. It's simply a non-issue for them.   If you are here, you already know or are at least in the "wondering" stage and this bears further investigating.   On the off chance that one of these nifty questionnaires hasn't been shoved in your face before now, here are just a few questions to ask yourself with regards to your alcohol and/or drug use that are "signs" of a problem (feel free to substitute the word "using" for "drinking" if that makes you feel better ...we aim to please):

- Not being able to quit drinking or control how much you drink
- Needing to drink more to feel the same effect
- Spending a lot of time drinking or to recover from drinking
- Giving up or forgoing activities so that you can drink instead
- Trying to quit drinking or cut down and not being able to
- Continuing to drink even after drinking has caused you problems
- Hiding, or trying to hide, your drinking from others
- Experiencing blackouts, where you don't remember events that happened while drinking
- Having friends, family, work, or others be concerned about your drinking

They say that, if you answer "Yes" to at least 3 of those questions, you probably have a problem with alcohol.   Most of the people that I know, myself included, probably answered a resounding "Hell Yes" to nearly every single one of those - and then went back out and continued to drink or drug until we were beaten down and thoroughly convinced that it was time to do something about it. Unfortunately, for an alcoholic or an addict to recover from this terrible disease (read Disease Chapter), they not only have to be convinced that they have it - easy enough for many - but they also have to be ready and willing to do something about it. Now there's a bit of a tall order. For all of us, this requires hitting some sort of "Bottom".

If we don't change our direction, we are likely to end up where we are headed - Ancient Chinese Proverb

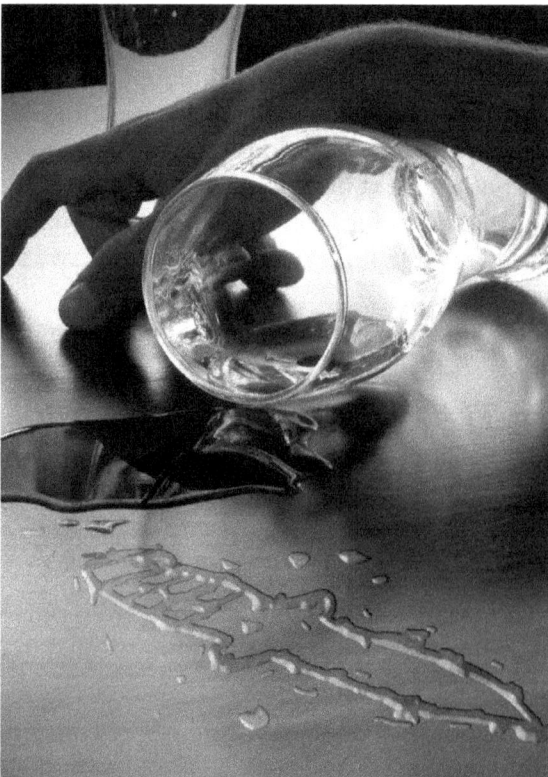

What's a Bottom?

When our myths, dreams, and ideals are shattered, our world topples. -Katherine Casey Thiesen

"Hitting Bottom" is a term that is heard over and over again with regards to people getting clean and sober - and for good reason. Most people are not willing to make changes without some pain and, let's face it, "pain is a great motivator". That's not to say that people's "bottom's" don't differ greatly and what is the final straw for you may not have phased me in the least to take a good hard look at myself. In fact, some of us are so resilient and "strong" that our bottoms will be many and they will continue to get lower and lower. Just to be clear: That was <u>not</u> a compliment.

Only an alcoholic thinks that they need to hit a lower bottom in order to be alcoholic. -sober alcoholic

A bottom for an alcoholic or addict can be many things but a lot of times arises from some bad situation as a result of drinking. Examples are DUIs, other arrests, losing a job (quitting right before you get fired is the same thing), losing friends, love interests, other financial consequences and so on. One popular saying about "bottoms" is that alcoholics hit their bottom when their losses pile up faster than they can lower their standards. We are great at justifying away the things that are slowly, or more quickly for others, marching out of our lives such as jobs, cars, houses, friends and family members. However, for some the turning point is more of an emotional bottom, where feelings of shame, loneliness, remorse and/or hopelessness become overwhelming and, despite still having the house, job, and cars in the garage, there comes a point where something has to change, and soon.

My personal experience was one of hitting many bottoms, where I suffered ever-increasing consequences as a result of my drinking and became acutely aware that something "had to change". However, for a very long time, I felt that the things that needed to change were the circumstances in my life. Things such as people, places, things and even the methods with which I went about drinking and using. I just wasn't "doing it right" and was still trying to figure out how to drink and drug the way I wanted to and not keep losing stuff or getting trouble.

Regardless if the circumstances of your life have brought you to your knees, it's become an unbearable internal struggle, or some combination of the two, it all comes down to a question of unmanageability. The simple fact of the matter is that the use of alcohol and/or drugs has become the ruling factor in my life and, in turn, my life has become a complete and utter shit storm. This is unmanageability at its finest and, if you can see this, you are well on your way to something much better. There is a lot to learn.

You never find yourself until you face the truth. -Pearl Bailey

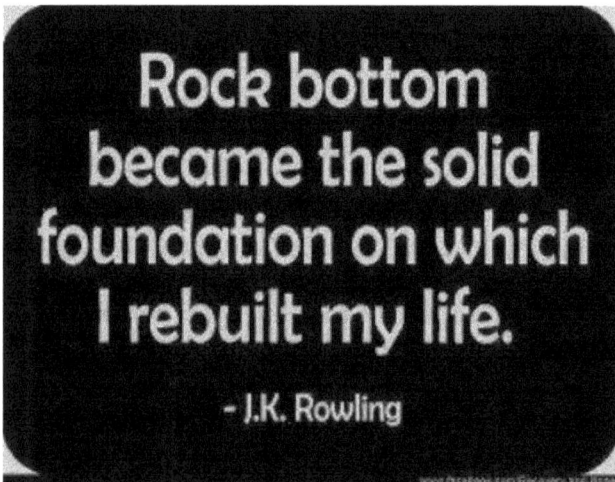

Rock bottom became the solid foundation on which I rebuilt my life.

- J.K. Rowling

Is Addiction Really a Disease?

"If I could drink like a regular person...I'd drink all the time. Therein lies our paradox..."

One fact that is both an unknown and a relief to many alcoholics is the fact that they actually have a "disease" and are not simply some social miscreant who cannot stop doing "wrong things". For over 100 years now, alcoholism has been widely known as, and treated as, a disease. In fact, in 1956, the American Medical Association voted to define alcoholism as a "disease". If you are in the midst of this maddening cycle, it will come as no surprise to you that drinking alcohol with regular frequency over time can produce a physical dependence on, or an addiction to, alcohol. Going a little deeper, however, we find out that drinking actually alters the balance of chemicals in your brain.

There is a chemical in your brain called glutamate, that serves to excite the nervous system. However, alcohol decreases glutamate's effectiveness, which is thought to be responsible for "memory blanks" and discoordination. GABA receptors, also in your brain, deal with impulsiveness. Alcohol can serve to enhance these functions, leading to anxiety reduction and loss of inhibition. Alcohol also raises the level of dopamine, which is the chemical that gives you that pleasurable feeling when you drink. Drugs like morphine or cocaine have been referred to as "chemical scalpels" because of their very precise effects on just one neurotransmitter system. Alcohol on the other hand is much more like a chemical hand grenade in that it affects just about all parts of the brain and all neurotransmitter systems. Chronic consumption of alcohol gradually makes the NMDA receptors hypersensitive to glutamate while desensitizing the GABAergic receptors. Making some sense now?

Some other disheartening facts are some of the contributing factors that may make you more predisposed to this disease. Things such as genetic predisposition and family history. In other words, you may be born with the "alcoholic gene" if this runs in your family and could be more predisposed to the behaviors if growing up in an alcoholic household. Age is a factor in that people who begin drinking and drugging at younger ages may be at higher risk. There also still seems to be a notion that alcoholism affects more men than women. Finally, emotional problems or disorders could also be factors that contribute to someone being at risk for developing this disease.

People who are prone to depression, anxiety and some emotional disorders may be more likely to turn to alcohol and drugs to regulate their moods. Recently, it has been thought that adults with ADHD may also be at higher risk. However, if these factors are "missing" in your "makeup", never fear. This does not preclude you from being an alcoholic. When I initially learned that this disease was "genetic", I turned heal and walked right back out the door as it does NOT run in my family. There is no doubt, however, that I do have this malady and was right where I needed to be.

A few characteristics of the Disease of Alcoholism (and Addiction) to be aware of are these:

Mental Obsession - Defined as a thought process over which you have no control. Sounds like fun, right? These maddening urges to drink, when many times we know that the results will be disastrous. I always call this the "preoccupation" that I always had with when I would be able to get that next drink or drug - or how I would be able to get more than my "share".

Chronic Disease - By chronic, we mean that it is "incurable" (keep reading anyway) and requires long-term treatment. This is a disease that can also result in death if not treated.

Progressive - This one is important. Well, the other two were also. Alcoholism is a subtly progressive disease that gets worse over time - NEVER better. Sometimes, this takes place over such an extended period of time that the alcoholic does not notice the point at which they truly lost control. And, you know what? It doesn't matter. Because as soon as that control is "lost", it can NEVER be regained. EVER. This is where the difficulty and the denial come into play for so many. We remember that time when things were great, fun, easy, controllable and try with all our might, sometimes for entirely too long, to recapture it. It just won't happen.

"Remember, once you're a pickle, you can never be a cucumber again."

The good news here is, you're sick! Bet you'd never considered putting something like that in your assets column, right? Think of it this way: You're not a bad person or an evil person that has crapped your life up. Rather, you're a "sick person" who simply needs to get well. And get well you can. While alcoholism isn't a disease that you can be cured of, it is one that you can recover from and lead a happy, healthy, productive life.

You are not responsible for your disease, but you are responsible for your behavior and, consequently, your recovery.

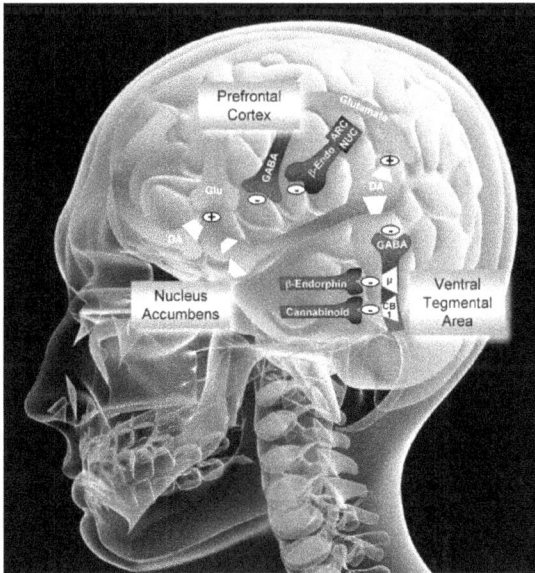

Taite Adams

Losing Everything - or Not

"...one of the primary differences between alcoholics and nonalcoholics is that nonalcoholics change their behavior to meet their goals and alcoholics change their goals to meet their behaviors." — *Alcoholics Anonymous*

There are many stories of people who have "recovered" from alcoholism who say that they "lost everything" to drugs and alcohol. But what does that mean, really? Honestly, that can be as subjective as the day is long. This comes down to several factors. One is - what is most important to you? If it's houses, cars, and boats - and those things start slipping away as a result of drinking, that may be enough to cry mercy and surrender. For others it's job or family that do the trick. Some have to lose their personal freedoms or have major health consequences to open their eyes. Finally, there are those who value peace of mind and self-respect above all else and raise the white flag as soon as they feel these things threatened as a result of their drinking or drugging activity.

My story is one of many "losses" as my disease and my stubbornness progressed at a breakneck pace. I lost some personal freedoms, material things, friends, jobs, and eventually even family as a result of my disease and my actions. All along the way, I was given multiple opportunities to throw in the towel and stop the madness. At every turn, I insisted there was "no problem" and that I knew exactly what I was doing and that things would be just fine if people would just leave me alone. It took losing nearly everything and the threat of losing my personal freedom for a very long time for me to finally give up fighting and try something else.

Unfortunately, a major characteristic of most alcoholics is extreme arrogance and stubbornness. Despite evidence to the contrary, ie- we are going to keep losing stuff at an ever increasing rate, we insist that we know best and want to give it one last college try to control this thing. Then, maybe just one more try. And so on. Many people view seeking help as a sign of weakness, yet refuse to see the forest for the trees by acknowledging the cold hard facts right in front of them - that they are being taken down a dark and dismal road of loss and heartache to which there is no happy ending without first getting some help. Despite hearing countless stories of people just like us who didn't stop and lost so much more, we insist this won't happen to us because "we're smarter" than that. When, in fact, the smarter of the bunch will get off that plummeting elevator right then and there and not have to lose another thing. The fact of the matter is this - we choose our bottom. This can be it - right now.

You don't have to be sick to want to get well. But if you don't want to get well, you ARE sick

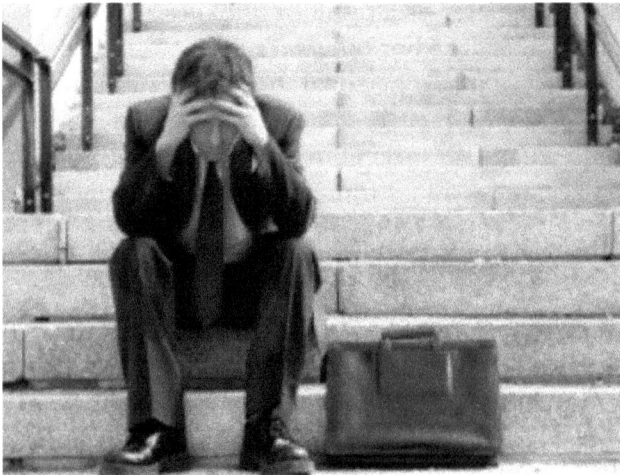

Detox Considerations

Every recovery from alcoholism and addiction begins with one sober hour.

It may sound obvious enough but it's the one thing that keeps many of us out there for much longer than necessary. Here it is: In order to stop drinking, you need to stop drinking. I know that I lived in fear of detox for years and this kept me scrambling to stay messed up enough on a continuous basis so that withdrawal symptoms didn't set in. What an awful way to live. Yes, detox is unpleasant, as it should be. By using drugs and alcohol to excess over an extended period of time, we have re-wired our bodies and minds to believe that those substances are "needed". While all instincts cry out that they most certainly are what is keeping us going, the truth is exactly the opposite. They are killing us.

In order to start the recovery process, detox is a must. Depending upon your drug of choice, the withdrawal symptoms and length of the detox are going to vary. Some people expect that they can attempt this at home. So many, in fact, that I have written an entirely separate book on How to Detox from Drugs and Alcohol at Home. This isn't always possible, or recommended, for a variety of reasons, however, so it is important that you do your homework before attempting this. Better yet, just check yourself into a medical detox facility and be done with it.

There are some substances that are very dangerous to detox from without medical supervision. These include, but are not limited to, alcohol and benzodiazepines. If you attempt self-detoxing with these substances, even with tapering (which isn't discussed in this book), you are taking great risks with your life. There are possibilities with other drugs but are beyond the scope of this book. Suffice to say that, if you are ready to quit and are sure that you have reached your bottom, ask for help.

Tips for Managing Cravings

Believe you can and you're halfway there. -Theodore Roosevelt

Whether you do a home detox, go to a medical detox, or try something else, it's very common in early recovery to have cravings. Cravings are urges to drink or use drugs. These urges are a normal part of any addiction and are common-place during withdrawal. They can also pop up months or even years after you stop using drugs.   Here are some important things to remember about cravings and some ways to deal with them.

What You Should Know About Cravings:

- They are not caused by a lack of willpower or motivation. It doesn't mean that you are doing something wrong or failing to do something right.
- Cravings don't mean that your detox and withdrawal aren't working.
- Cravings pass. These urges are not constant and are only severe for a very short period of time before they settle down to a more controllable level.
- Cravings can be triggered by physical or psychological discomfort. Managing these can help manage the onset and severity of cravings.

Things You Can Do to Manage Cravings:

- Remind yourself that cravings are "temporary". In fact, if the urge to use is very strong, simply put the decision off for an hour and the feelings will likely subside.
- Identify cues or "triggers" that may have brought on the cravings. They could people, places or things that remind you

of using. Re-direct your mental energy towards ways in which you can avoid these same triggers in the future.

- Remind yourself of why you stopped taking the drug in the first place. This would be the time to re-list the negative effects that the drug use had on your life and also list the positive things that you stand to gain by staying clean.
- Call on others for help. This is where a Support Network comes in, supportive family members and friends that support your recovery.
- Use your spirituality to get through cravings. Prayer and meditation can help calm the mind and bring focus back into what you have achieved so far and what lies ahead in your recovery.

Now that we've covered some basic things to know about detoxing, let's explore what needs to be done afterwards in order to remain clean and begin a life of recovery from addiction.

Should I Go to Treatment?

If you want what you've never had, you must do what you've never done.

This is a tough question to answer and highly debated. If you spend any time watching television (most do), then many just assume that to "get sober", you have to go to treatment. This isn't necessarily the case. Historically, men and women have been getting and staying sober without the help of fancy treatment centers. Many people are able to get sober and stay sober with the help of 12 Step programs alone - no rehab. They simply walk into AA one day, "get started" and never have to pick up a drink or a drug again. However, in our fast-paced society with all of life's demands, treatment centers have certainly carved out a solid slot in the "getting sober" process for many over the years and have very real value.

Honestly, many of you may not have a choice. Treatment centers have become the "sentence" of choice for many criminal and family courts in recent years. Get yourself into any sort of jackpot even remotely related to drugs or alcohol and, next thing you know, it's off to treatment in lieu of serving time and paying fines. I know that my tour of the treatment center circuit started courtesy of the courts. Regardless of your circumstances, here is some information to help you make a more informed decision about "checking in" or not. And, if so, where?

Kickstart Your Recovery

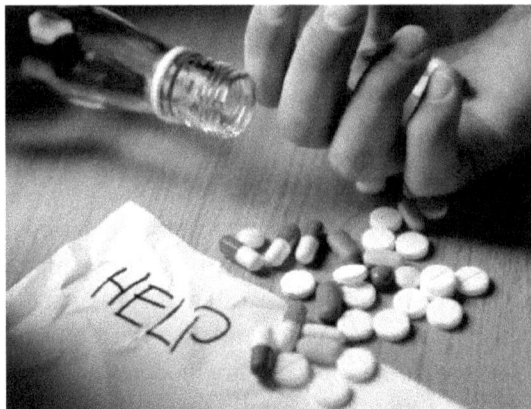

Not All Treatment Centers Are the Same

...we do not always like what is good for us in this world. -Eleanor Roosevelt

There are many, many different types of rehabs out there and the choices can be very confusing. However, let's take a look at what many of them have in common before we get to the differences. According to the **National Survey of Substance Abuse Treatment Services**, there is a certain "formula" for a successful treatment program that has become somewhat standard. This includes:

- **Assessment and Evaluation** - This includes both physical and psychological evaluation to determine where you are at, gather history information, and develop current diagnoses.

- **Alcohol/Drug Detox** - This refers to the time after which the body stops taking in alcohol and drugs and will, probably, undergo some withdrawal symptoms. Medical care for these issues is provided.

- **Counseling and therapeutic treatment** - After detox, "treatment" starts that involves both counseling from certified counselors and support from other recovering alcoholics.

- **Aftercare** - Ongoing support through personal and group therapies, 12 step meetings and other holistic treatments.

Now, all of that being similar, choices abound as to what sort of treatment center, if any, is going to be right for you. You will need to decide between Inpatient or Outpatient, Private or Public and, in some cases, Co-Ed or Single Sex treatment centers. For example, I've been to a private outpatient co-ed treatment center, a private inpatient co-ed treatment center, a public outpatient same-sex treatment center and a public inpatient co-ed treatment center, just to name a few.

Inpatient vs Outpatient

Many people are inclined to select "outpatient" right off the bat because we are also inclined to downplay the seriousness of our situation and the means necessary to recover from it. This is what I did. I went through quite a few outpatient treatment programs and they served several purposes for me. They got the courts off my back to an extent, they educated me about my disease and they allowed me to continue to pretend to manage my life on the "outside" for a little bit longer while I racked up some more consequences and losses. Some people are able to successfully participate in treatment programs on a part-time basis while continuing to live at home, manage their family lives and keep their jobs. These people are exceptions to the rule, however. There are other outpatient treatment programs that simply have you go to treatment during the day and return to your home (and family) at night. Again, depending on your circumstances, this may be a viable option. For many, and for a lot of reasons, it's not for the majority of people.

Inpatient drug and alcohol treatment is more the norm for quite a few reasons. This option dictates that the individual moves into some sort of dorm-like setting and receives 24/7 care and supervision. Some treatment centers allow for private and semi-private rooms, while others dictate that you will essentially take what you are given. Inpatient treatment is the ideal choice for someone who needs a place to focus entirely on their addiction and developing their recovery program.

Private vs Public

Regardless of the previous differences, you will run into rehab centers that are both Private and Publicly funded. Different treatment funding sources include:

- Private: Non-profit, or For Profit
- State or Locally Funded
- Low Cost Treatment Centers
- Free Rehabs (Charity Rehabs)

While the Free, Low Cost and Government Funded treatment centers sound great (they are, I got sober in one), it's important to note that many also have long waiting lists. You may even need to get onto a long waiting list to get into a publicly-funded detox facility. Another difference, although not true in all cases, may be the size of groups in therapy sessions, with smaller groups in Private facilities and larger groups in publicly funded rehabs. Also, do not expect to get into any sort of private or semi-private room in a public facility. In retrospect, being "pampered" did nothing to get me sober. I did find the many waiting lists very disheartening, though, when I was finally "ready" for this and just couldn't get in anyplace. So, if you are looking at Private treatment centers and possible ways to finance it, consider these:

- **Health Insurance** - most "good" health insurance policies provide for some form of substance abuse treatment. If you have a really good policy, you may be able to get an inpatient treatment program paid for
- **Family Members** - you may already have family members offering to pay to get you sober. I did. I even had friends of family willing to chip in at one point.
- **Sell stock or take money from your 401k** - If you're unemployed, in jail or dead, there will be no "retirement" to save for, right?
- **Home Equity Loan** - If you are lucky enough to still be holding onto your home, consider this.
- **Sell stuff, even your car** - Chances are you have expensive toys you haven't been using because of you've been putting all of your efforts into drinking and drugging. Sell them. You don't need a car if you're not sober. It's a hazard.
- **Substance Abuse Treatment Loan** - Yes, they have these now.

Co-ed vs Same Sex Treatment Centers

I've been to both and it didn't make a difference to me either way. However, if you have been the victim of abuse and think that you would feel safer in a same sex facility, by all means, check them out. Otherwise, you will find just as many people at both types of facilities that want to get sober, that don't want to get sober, or are looking for other sorts of distractions.

The Pro's and Con's of Going to Treatment

I have found that sitting in a place where you have never sat before can be inspiring.
-Dodie Smith

When I first started hitting the treatment centers, I didn't see any "Pro's" whatsoever. I did not want to be there, did not think that I had a problem like the rest of the folks in that place did and felt very inconvenienced by the whole thing. Quite a few treatment centers and many years of sobriety later, it's much easier to see their benefit. However, I do clearly see what the Con's are in committing to these institutions. Here are a few:

Con's of Going to Treatment

Time - Yes, you are committing a substantial amount of your time to this program. You are committing literally ALL of your time if you elect to go to an inpatient treatment center. This means that family and work responsibilities need to be re-arranged. In many cases, some or all of those have "dissolved" on their own because of our drinking and drugging activities.

Cost - Most people would agree that this is the biggest downside to treatment, particularly private rehabs. Inpatient programs can cost upwards of $1,000 per day and outpatient programs are not cheap either. Publicly funded programs are more affordable but there are oftentimes many hoops to jump through to qualify and get into these programs.

Pro's of Going to Treatment

Structured Environment - One of the biggest benefits of attending treatment, primarily residential (or inpatient), is that you are provided with a safe, structured environment that is free of distractions and temptations. This will give you a window of opportunity to Kickstart Your Recovery, get sober and learn how to live life without drugs and alcohol. This structured environment is designed to essentially be free of the daily stressors of work, home and family so that you can focus only on your recovery.

Establish Network of Positive People - Attending treatment, inpatient or outpatient, gives you the opportunity to form new friendships and bonds with other like-minded, positive people. These are relationships that can be the beginning of your sober support network.

Learning Better Holistic Health - If giving up drinking and drugs were enough, this would be a much shorter book. However, the real purpose of recovery is to learn how to live a happy and healthy life without drugs and alcohol. Learning to treat yourself well in all respects is something that you can learn in treatment, such as eating right, being physically active and taking care of your mental and spiritual well-being.

Save Money - Wait, what?! Didn't we just say in the "Con's" that "cost" was a downside to going to treatment? Well, yes we did. BUT, let's look at the big picture here. The amount of money that you will save in long run by getting, and staying sober, is astounding compared to continuing with that financial minefield of active addiction. Many people are blown away when they see the financial figures tied to their disease. I'm not just talking about the money spent on drugs and alcohol (count this, though). Add in jobs lost, promotions lost, missed opportunities, legal fees, smashed cars, foreclosed homes, and so on. Looking at it this way, the cost of a stint at that fancy rehab may not look as outrageous as it did earlier.

Save Your Life - For some, it really does boil down to this. It's simply a matter of life or death. Without some real, structured help, the end is imminent. A lot of addicts and alcoholics run to treatment in hopes that they will "save" something or get their lives back. What many find is that they have been given an entirely new life that is infinitely better than anything they could have ever dreamed possible.

At fifteen life had taught me undeniably that surrender, in its place, was as honorable as resistance, especially if one had no choice. -Maya Angelou

IF IT IS IMPORTANT TO YOU, YOU WILL FIND A WAY. IF NOT, YOU'LL FIND AN EXCUSE.

If You Decide To Go

All glory comes from daring to begin. -Eugene F. Ware

If you make the decision to go to a treatment facility, good for you! You are giving yourself a gift that will not only come back to you tenfold but to those you know and love as well, even if they aren't speaking to you right now.

As I stated before, there are so many different types of treatment facilities so it's not possible to give you a perfect run down of what to expect. However, here are a few standards and a few words of wisdom:

There will be no locks on the doors. This doesn't work, not even for a second, if you're not willing so you can walk away at any time. Even if you are court ordered to be at a place, they'll just come and pick you up to face your consequences at a later date should you bolt. Check your willingness level at the door, and thereafter frequently, and commit to stay for whatever term is recommended.

You may be entering a detox facility first that is either separate or affiliated with the treatment center. This can last anywhere from 2-7 days and, while not pleasant, is absolutely necessary before anything else can take place to help you. You will be given medication to ease the negative effects of the withdrawals and probably just sleep a lot. Remember, you never have to do this again.

The rehab center itself will be different, depending on where you go. However, after detox, expect to "check in" and get situated with lodgings and a schedule. Just remember, the "posh factor" of your particular rehab facility, ie- whether you get your own room (not likely), are near a beach, have a pool, etc., has absolutely nothing to do with how successful this place will be in getting you clean and sober. The main factor here is you and your attitude. If you walk into this place willing to "go to any lengths" to get sober, you will.

The education and counseling will likely start right away. Both are key components to any successful treatment program. Expect to be educated on the disease of alcoholism, including the physical effects of your addiction and what is going to happen should you continue to use. Daily group therapy sessions are the norm as well as periodic individual counseling with a trained addictions counselor. These sessions cover many things but center on breaking through denial, teaching skills to live life without drugs and alcohol, and relapse prevention.

Family meetings are also often part of a rehab program, wherein family and/or friends are invited in to learn about addiction and to participate in family counseling sessions. Finally, Aftercare Programs are also common, where a strong plan is developed for "after" treatment, that may involve outpatient treatment, counseling, residence at a halfway house, periodic "check ins" with your counselor and other suggestions to help avoid triggers and relapse. Nearly all successful rehab facilities and aftercare plans are going to incorporate 12 Step meetings into their curriculum. This means that you will more than likely be going to nightly AA (or NA) meetings from the treatment center and be recommended to continue with these when you leave.

If you go - From my experience with the revolving doors of many treatment centers, these are my words of wisdom. First and foremost, check the attitude at the door. This is one thing that I took in with me and held onto through nearly all of my stays, except for the last one. It did me no favors. Thinking that I still knew what was best for me, after the shit storm that I had just made of my life was ludicrous. Also, demanding that I be given respect and attention when I felt I needed it was just as insane. I had to come to a place where I finally understood that I knew absolutely nothing about how to recover from this disease and that these people were clearly authorities on the subject. So probably, I should just let them do their job and listen to someone else for a change. Once I did this - made this mental shift (some would call it "surrender"), going to treatment was a blessing for me and I made the most of every single opportunity that was put in front of me to learn and to start my recovery. Yes, this included going to AA, which I also resisted for a long time.

The significant problems we have cannot be solved at the same level of thinking with which we created them. -Albert Einstein

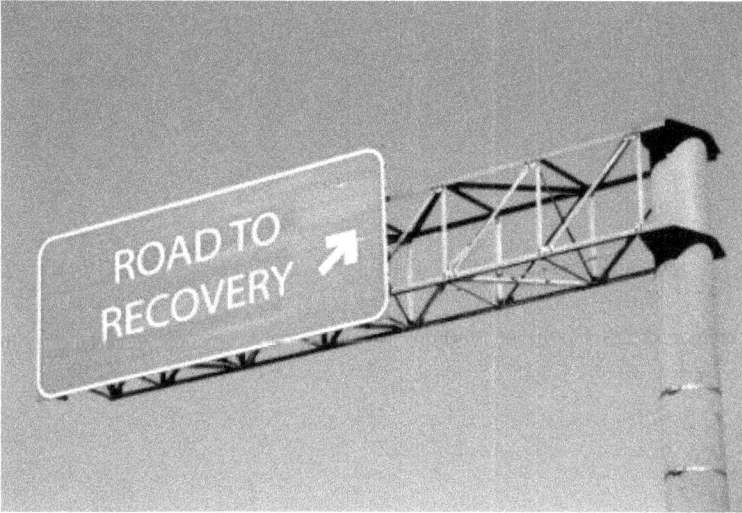

What is AA?

"The feeling of having shared in a common peril is one element in the powerful cement which binds us." — Alcoholics Anonymous

Many people, myself included, have avoided getting sober simply because they feared "joining" AA. I had no concept of what this group was or just how something like this could possibly be of any assistance to me. I didn't understand what AA was and there is always the fear of the unknown. So, what is AA then? Well, if you ask them:

Alcoholics Anonymous® is a fellowship of men and women who share their experience, strength and hope with each other that they may solve their common problem and help others to recover from alcoholism. The only requirement for membership is a desire to stop drinking. There are no dues or fees for AA membership; we are self-supporting through our own contributions. AA is not allied with any sect, denomination, politics, organization or institution; does not wish to engage in any controversy, neither endorses nor opposes any causes. Our primary purpose is to stay sober and help other alcoholics to achieve sobriety

What it is, really, is a multi-faceted program that incorporates meetings, fellowship and working a 12-step program in order to bring about a change in the alcoholic and provide continued growth and support. AA was founded in 1935 by Bill Wilson (known as Bill W) and Dr. Robert Smith (known as Dr. Bob), based on the main principle of one alcoholic sharing their experiences with another. Within 4 years, their basic text called "Alcoholics Anonymous" (aka The Big Book) was published and membership blossomed. Today, there are over 2 million members of AA world-wide (over 1/2 of these in the U.S.) and over 115,000 registered AA Groups. In fact, there are now over 200 different fellowships that employ the "12 Steps" for recovery from AA (altered to fit). Hard to argue with those numbers.

Separate reeds are easily broken; but bound together they are strong and hard to break apart. -The Midrash

Kickstart Your Recovery

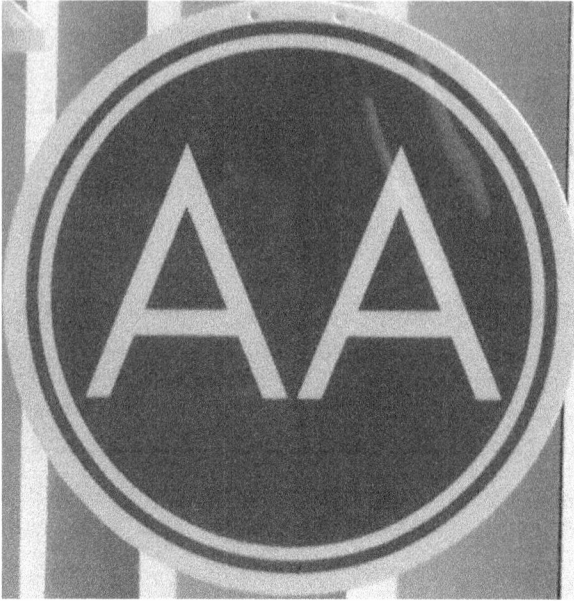

Taite Adams

Is AA a Cult?

The circle stands for the whole world of A.A., and the triangle stands for A.A.'s Three Legacies of Recovery, Unity, and Service.

There are SO many websites that will debate this point, that I don't really need to get too deep into it here. However, it is an often asked question by newcomers and is sometimes mentioned at meetings (tongue in cheek, or not). The answer? Ummm ...it could be, sort of. Who in their right mind said when they were a kid - "hey, I want to grow up to be an addict or an alcoholic and then join a cult to get better?" Uh - I don't recall ever uttering those words. However, there is no disputing that AA works and is, hands down, the most successful program for achieving and maintaining sobriety. Are there some "cultish" elements at work here? Perhaps. Charlie Sheen ranted on Twitter that AA is nothing but "a Cult of stupid people". Now, who's going to argue with the likes of Charlie Sheen?

A cult is defined as a group of people who have divine faith in a person, belief, object or movement. What separates a cult from recognized religious organizations is that the term is used in reference to a group or organization with practices and beliefs that are considered abnormal or bizarre. Cults serve diverse purposes for individuals, including a positive sense of community with defined values. Cults offer acceptance, unconditional love and support as well as a strong sense of family within the group. For those who have been through a difficult life filled with harm, sadness and abuse, these organizations can be everything that they had hoped and dreamed of. Can you get these things in AA? Yes, you absolutely can. But I got many of them on my water polo team, too.

Thomas Lynch, in an article on beliefnet.com called "AA: Not Religious, Not a Cult," says this about AA: *My church, my Rotary club, and my bowling league are each more cultish than A.A. is. It takes no tithes, commissions, fines, or fees. There's no kool-aid to drink, communion to take, secret codes, or insignia. A.A. does not work by shame or guilt or fear or pride or power. It works by surrender, letting go, giving up, listening. It does not promise salvation, justice, fortune, or a better figure. You may come and go as you please. It claims no corner on the market of God. In fact, the only article of faith it requires is that if there's a God, it isn't me.*

Critics of the Big Book compare its text to the religious texts of other cults. It represents stories, lessons and guidelines for people who are overcoming alcoholism in a simple way and say it provides stories to explain the faults of non-believers. This is one perspective. Other critics see AA as having an element of "Separatism" to it, where members see themselves as outsiders and different from the rest of society. This also sometimes leads to separate language or "jargon" that only members understand. Charismatic leaders are characteristic of most cults and, while AA's tend to be a bit "in awe" of their founders, those guys have been dead for many years and the organization has no effective "leadership" whatsoever in the present day.

True story: In my first year of sobriety myself and my best friend Michelle were invited to an AA movie "get together" on a Saturday night. We met a group of AA members at this room in the back of a warehouse to watch an old, historic, interview film of Bill W., one of the founders of AA. Everyone brought food and snacks. The two of us were standing outside during a break, looking in at this group of people - lined up, sitting at tables in the dark, drinking tea and juice, and watching an old black and white video of our (dead) "leader". I looked at my friend and said "holy shit, Michelle. We've joined a goddamn cult!". She said, "uh huh". And we both went back inside and sat down for the second half.

Here's the thing. Cult, no cult. It works. It's really more "no cult" than it is otherwise anyway. And by the time we get here, each and every one of us could use a serious brain washing, and then rinse and repeat. Consider these final thoughts before moving on. If AA is a cult it has to be one of the oddest cults of all; Think about it, how many cults have you heard of that:

1. You can believe, or not believe, in a higher power of your choice.
2. You can quit with no backlash from members.
3. You can quit and come back as often as you like with no backlash from members.

4. You can follow the suggestions if you wish or not.
5. You can attend drunk as a skunk for years.
6. You can put money in the basket or not.
7. There are no rules.

A.A. is no success story in the ordinary sense of the word. It is a story of suffering transmuted, under grace, into spiritual progress. AS BILL SEES IT, p. 35

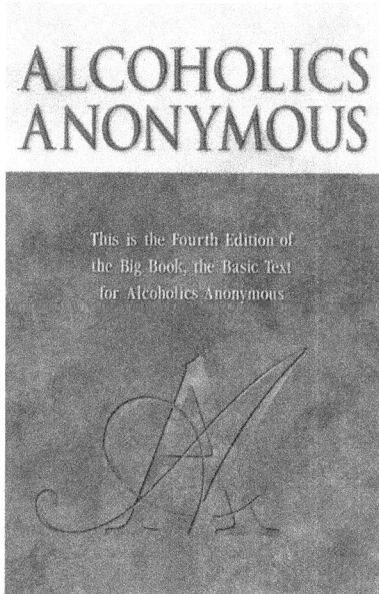

But...How Does it Work?

"Shared joy is double joy, and shared sorrow is half-sorrow." -Swedish Proverb

For years, I took issue with these treatment centers, "recovery programs" and 12 step meetings that threw what I saw as a bunch of hocus pocus stuff up in front of me and told me that if I would only give it a try, I would be "well on my way" to getting better. I didn't get it. I was educated and pretty smart, dammit, and I wanted someone to spell out for me in black and white just HOW doing those things was going to help me. That's a tough order.

What I found was that I had to get to a place of desperation and complete willingness, where I just didn't care "How" it worked anymore. I just knew for a fact, finally, that my way wasn't working and was willing to try something else. This giving up of control is a big step for anyone, but especially so for someone in the throes of addiction. Recovery from alcoholism happens on many levels: physical, mental, emotional and spiritual. The program of AA addresses these different levels of recovery through its different facets of: attending meetings, getting a sponsor, working the 12 steps, spiritual principles and involvement in the fellowship.

In doing these things, old habits are broken, new (healthy) habits are formed, and we are able to take a deeper look at the causes and conditions underlying our long drinking careers. All of this is done in some manner that taps into the mechanisms that counter the complex neurological and psychological processes through which this disease wreaks its havoc. Better yet, it's done through the power of "the group". Psychologists have long known that one of the best ways to change human behavior is to gather people with similar problems into groups instead of treating them individually. This is one of AA's precepts.

Whether it is the initial act of "surrender", the group support setting, the self-awareness that comes from working the Steps, or the close relationships in the fellowship through helping others that are the key components to the alcoholic's recovery (one or all of these), no one knows. What we do know, however, is that despite all we've learned over the past few decades about psychology, neurology, and human behavior, contemporary medicine has yet to devise anything that works markedly better. "In my 20 years of treating addicts, I've never seen anything else that comes close to the 12 steps," says Drew Pinsky, the addiction-medicine specialist who hosts VH1's Celebrity Rehab. "In my world, if someone says they don't want to do the 12 steps, I know they aren't going to get better." As we continue to study and collect data, a growing body of evidence suggests that, while AA may not be a miracle cure for all, people who become deeply involved in the program stay sober and do well over the long haul, and this starts with attending meetings.

We perceive that only through utter defeat are we able to take our first steps toward liberation and strength. Our admissions of personal powerlessness finally turn out to be firm bedrock upon which happy and purposeful lives may be built. TWELVE STEPS AND TWELVE TRADITIONS, p. 21

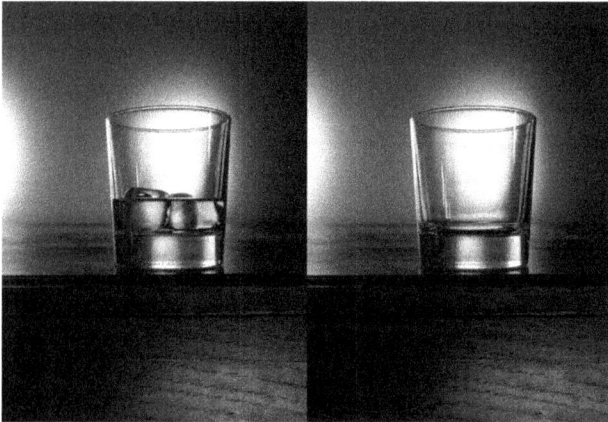

The Meetings

There were deep secrets, hidden in my heart, never said for fear others would scoff or snear. At last I can reveal my sufferings, for the strength I once felt in silence has lost all its power. -Deidra Sarault

Everything about getting sober is uncomfortable, sometimes painful and just plain weird. Attendance at your first AA meetings fits in nicely with that. No one feels completely "at ease" walking into their first AA meeting. Most people are completely petrified, horrified or just plain angry at the thought that this is where they've ended up. One useful thing to remember is that, despite the many happy faces you will see in the room (more on that later), every single person there had the very same experience that you are having and you are not alone. Don't dismiss a meeting just because you think it's weird (it may be) or because you didn't understand anything that went on there. Give it a chance. Go to several meeting and several different kinds of meetings before passing judgment. Yes, AA meetings are a bit ritualistic and have a "format". Here is a little bit about what you can expect at a typical meeting:

AA Meetings are held in many different sorts of places. Oftentimes, they are held in churches, schools, and other public buildings. You can find nearly any meeting list online by just googling "aa meetings" and your town. If you arrive early, you will likely find people standing outside talking and smoking, as most meetings are now non-smoking. Usually, there is coffee available at meetings and sometimes cookies or snacks. AA meetings generally last an hour and are pretty punctual with their starting and ending times. A meeting will be run by a "Chairperson", who will lead a meeting for a week, a month, or a specified period and then someone else will take over the position. This person simply "leads" or facilitates the meeting, they are not in charge.

When a meeting starts, the Chairperson will call the meeting to order. There is generally a moment of Silence followed by the Serenity Prayer

("God, grant me the serenity to accept the things I cannot change, the courage to change the things I can, and the wisdom to know the difference"). Sometimes there are additional readings from the Big Book, such as "How it Works" and other items that the chairperson needs to read. The Chairperson will also ask if there is anyone attending their first AA meeting or if there is anyone "New". This is your cue if you wish to raise your hand and just say your name. You don't have to give a speech (please, don't). They just want your name - nothing else. The Chairperson will also, at some point, ask if there is anyone "having a problem staying sober today"? This is also an opportunity for you to raise your hand, say your name again, and let people know that you are having a tough time - if you are.

The meeting will then continue depending upon the meeting format. At some point, the meeting will pause for a basket to be passed. This is AA's 7th Tradition that states that the program is "self-supporting". Many people put in $1 into the basket. Do not feel pressured to put anything into the basket at all until you are more comfortable going to the meetings, or until your financial situation dictates. At the end of the meeting, or at some point before, chips will be handed out. Chips are handled differently at every meeting but most meetings give out a "white chip", which is the universal sign of surrender. If this is your first meeting and you wish to "surrender" and join, go up and pick up a white chip. If you aren't ready to do this yet, that's ok. Keep coming back. At the end of the meeting, group members will stand and join hands to say either the Lord's Prayer or the Serenity Prayer, for those who care to.

These are the basic meeting elements that you will encounter regardless of the meeting format or where you attend meetings. This allows members to walk into any meeting, anyplace in the world and feel "at home", even if the meeting is taking place in another language.

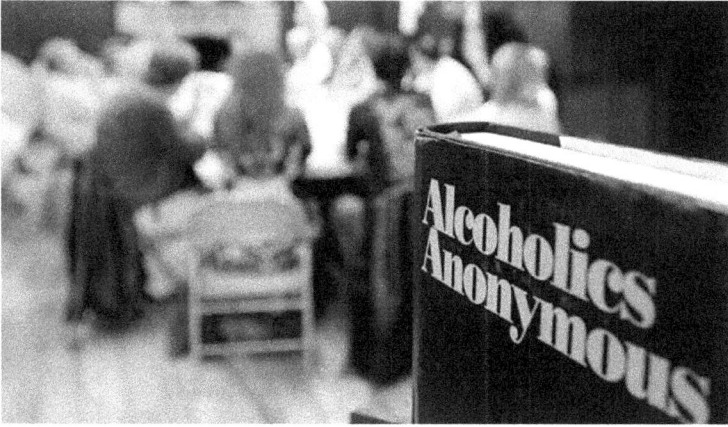

Meeting Formats

You may already have asked yourself why it is that all of us became so very ill from drinking. Doubtless you are curious to discover how and why, in the face of expert opinion to the contrary, we have recovered from a hopeless condition of mind and body. If you are an alcoholic who wants to get over it, you may already be asking-- "What do I have to do?" -Alcoholics Anonymous, p. 20

Now that we have the elements of an AA Meeting down (what you will find at every meeting), what about the Formats? Meeting formats change. There are quite a few different types of AA Meetings. On the one hand, this can be confusing to the newcomer. On the other hand, it keeps things fresh and interesting for those who like to attend various types of meetings.

Open vs Closed Meetings - First and foremost, every meeting will either be an Open Meeting or a Closed Meeting. Open Meetings are "open" for attendance to anyone. This means that anyone who thinks that they may have a problem with drinking, someone who is supporting an alcoholic, someone who is "just curious", physicians and academics are free to attend these meetings. Closed Meetings are just that - They are only open to people who have a desire to stop drinking. If you are wondering whether you are an alcoholic or not, attend either. I can tell you that there is no ticket taker at the door conducting interviews to determine whether you "belong" there or not. If you think you do, you most certainly do.

Discussion Meetings - The chairperson will bring up a topic, either from their personal experience in recovery or from AA approved literature, and then open up discussion to the rest of the group.
Speaker Meetings - Another member of AA, generally with 6 months or more of sobriety, will tell their story to the group. If there is time after the speaker finishes, discussion may be opened up to the group.
Big Book Meetings - Passages or a chapter from the Big Book is read and other members then comment on that passage and how it relates to their recovery.

Step Study Meetings - This is the same idea as the Big Book meeting but the text used is the "Twelve Steps and Twelve Traditions" or "12 and 12". Members read and then share with respect to the passages read.

Beginner Meetings - Focus on people with less than one year of sobriety, who are given the opportunity to share on a topic. Discussion is opened up to "old timers" afterwards if there is time. (Definitely search out and attend some of these).

Other Meetings - There are quite a few meeting formats (too many to list). A few other are Living Sober Meetings (another literature study), Grapevine Meetings (AA Magazine study), Women's Meetings (Women Only), Men's Meetings (Men Only), YPG (Young People's Group - anyone is welcome here), and so on.

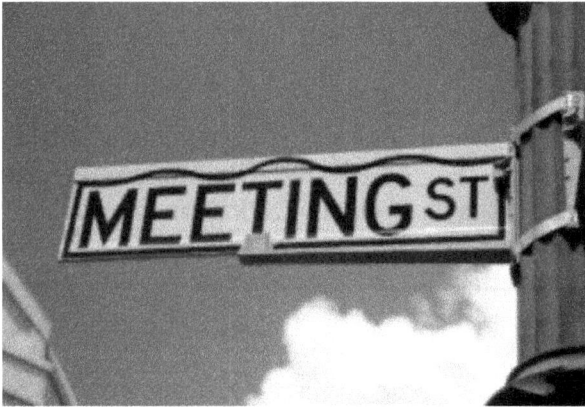

HOW Many Meetings?

Newcomers are often horrified when they hear the recommendation that they attend 90 Meetings in 90 Days (aka "90 in 90"). This is, of course, a "recommendation" or a suggestion and not a requirement for membership. This came about from the realization that the people who made it 90 days without a relapse had a much better chance of sustained recovery and that the 90-day point represented some sort of threshold. A recent Time Magazine article goes on to say *"... It turns out that this is just about how long it takes for the brain to reset itself and shake off the immediate influence of a drug. Researchers at Yale University have documented what they call the sleeper effect--a gradual re-engaging of proper decision making and analytical functions in the brain's prefrontal cortex--after an addict has abstained for at least 90 days."* There are many benefits to, number one - taking suggestions and number two - actually doing the 90 meetings in 90 days.

First, by actually taking the suggestion and making this commitment, the individual is showing that they are really willing to change their life and willingness is a key element to obtaining and sustaining sobriety. A big part of it is the "exposure" that you get to the program that allows you to learn how the program works, get some support and meet some new people. This also ensures that the program becomes a priority and can be a great self-esteem boost and confidence boost simply because you are keeping a daily commitment. Honestly, this was not an issue for me in early sobriety. I was sufficiently willing, freaked out and humbled enough to do whatever was asked of me and I spent far more than an hour a day drinking, drugging and suffering the consequences of those actions. This didn't seem too much to ask and I often went to several meetings a day to pass the time and get to know people.

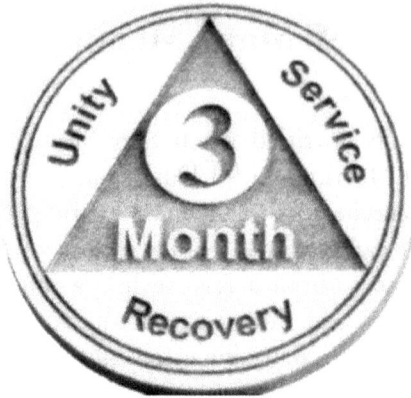

A few other important things to cover about AA Meetings are: the all important Meeting Etiquette, the importance of a Home Group, the role of AA Clubs and Clubhouses and Alternative Meeting Formats.

Meeting Etiquette

Almost without exception, alcoholics are tortured by loneliness. Even before our drinking got bad and people began to cut us off, nearly all of us suffered the feeling that we didn't quite belong. AS BILL SEES IT, p. 90

Whether you are walking into your first AA meeting or your twentieth, the process can still be intimidating and, as a newcomer, new coping skills have yet to be developed to help ease the pain. I know that I like to have a good idea about what I'm about to walk into and how I should "act", so here are some general guidelines about meeting etiquette so that you can feel slightly more at ease.

First, relax. Nothing is that big of a deal and, despite your best efforts to the contrary, the people in the rooms of AA will be able to spot a newcomer a mile away. No one should put you on the spot and you will always be made to feel welcome. If anyone ever asks you to say anything and you simply don't want to, the standard reply is "I'd just like to listen" or "I'll pass". That's it - moving on.

A common tactic used by many to reduce anxiety and avoid having to speak to anyone is to arrive late to the meeting and leave early. Don't do this as you are selling yourself short. If you have social anxiety, as most of us do, simply use the few minutes before the meeting to grab a cup of coffee and check out some of the free literature that is laid out. In time, that unease will lessen. Here are some other etiquette guidelines to keep in mind:

- Turn off your cell phone! - Don't put it on "vibrate" and don't text, surf the web or email people during the meeting. Just silence the thing and put it away. Most meetings will announce this at the beginning to remind you.
- If you speak, identify yourself - At the very least, give your name. You can say, "Hi, My name is Joe" or "My name is Joe, I'm an alcoholic". Up to you. But, members expect to hear your name before they hear anything else from you.

- No "Double Dipping" - This means that if you share in a meeting, that's it. You don't get to raise your hand and share again later. (There are exceptions to this rule for some literature study meeting formats).
- Limit your comments to no more than 3 minutes. You will notice other members breaking this "guideline" constantly. Trust me - stick to it and you will be hailed and respected.
- No "Cross Talking" - This refers to directly addressing another member when you speak (or share) or directly addressing the comments of another member.
- Never interrupt someone who is speaking or be disruptive by talking, or whispering, to your neighbor (aka "side conversations").
- When sharing, talk about personal experiences and feelings as they relate to recovery and the meeting topic. This is generally referred to as sharing your "experience, strength and hope". It is not cool, ever, to tell another member what to think or how to behave. This isn't about giving or getting "advice", rather identification and sharing of similar experiences and feelings in recovery. This may sound confusing. If so, simply sit back and observe for a bit and you will get the idea.

Finally, just keep coming back. What may seem foreign, stifling and even very strange in the beginning provides an odd sense of comfort once you begin to become accustomed to it. And remember, none of us walked into the rooms of AA for the first time understanding any of this stuff. While there appear to be a lot of "rules", there really aren't any. These are simply guidelines to follow for groups of people who are used to living their lives by no rules whatsoever. We are people from all walks of life with a common problem who come together to learn how to get well and to start respecting ourselves and each other.

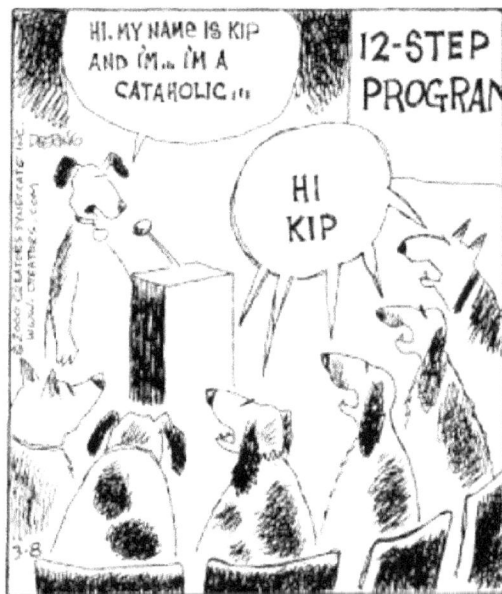

The Home Group

We recovered alcoholics are not so much brothers in virtue as we are brothers in our defects, and in our common strivings to overcome them AS BILL SEES IT, p. 167

The term is used often, either in treatment centers, at beginner meetings, or just generally read in some meeting formats, but no one really stops to explain what exactly a "Home Group" in AA is. You are simply told that you should "get" one, yet there is no guide as to how to go about doing this either. Or why you should at all.

The "Home Group" actually stems from AAs roots, where early members would meet in the "homes" of fellow members. From these "Home Groups", they would go out to help newcomers seeking sobriety through AA. As AA has grown, and meetings became held in public venues, the concept of the Home Group still held true. This group becomes your "home base", if you will, and will be the meeting that you make a commitment to attend as often as you are able. As a member of a Home Group, you then have the right and privilege to vote in that group's business meetings and to participate in the AA service structure through that group (there are other service opportunities not tied to the group, however).

AA members are members of AA as a whole in any given meeting, anyplace in the world. However, in their Home Group, they are also members of that group. In general, it will be the place where they celebrate their AA Anniversary as well as where members form the strongest bonds with other members. For many, this becomes an extended family and strong friendships are formed. It also adds a layer of accountability to your recovery, wherein members will take notice if you stop attending or seem to have something bothering you (this is a good thing).

Another advantage of being a member of a Home Group and attending regularly is that you have a group of people who really get to know you well and become "invested" in your life and your trials.

They will visit you in the hospital, call when you lose a loved one and offer advice when you ask them for it. I remember being a few years sober and struggling with how to break my anonymity to my boss. I was in a situation where it had to be done. I had members of my home group that would ask me every week, "Taite, what's going on with your work situation?". (It turned out fine). That was nice to have other people that cared enough to be thinking about my problems, wanting to help, and wanting a positive outcome for me.

As far as how to "join" a Home Group goes, it may be as simple as saying (to yourself), "this is my home group". That is how my current home group operates. It's your "Home Group" if you say it is. Others, you simply sign your first name in a book and you're "in". It's that simple. If in doubt, simply ask the Chairperson after a meeting and they will be glad to help you. In general, most people are members of just one Home Group.

Over the years, the very essence of A.A. strength has remained with our home group, which, for many members, becomes our extended family. Once isolated by our drinking, we find in the home group a solid, continuing support system, friends and, very often, a sponsor. -Alcoholics Anonymous World Services

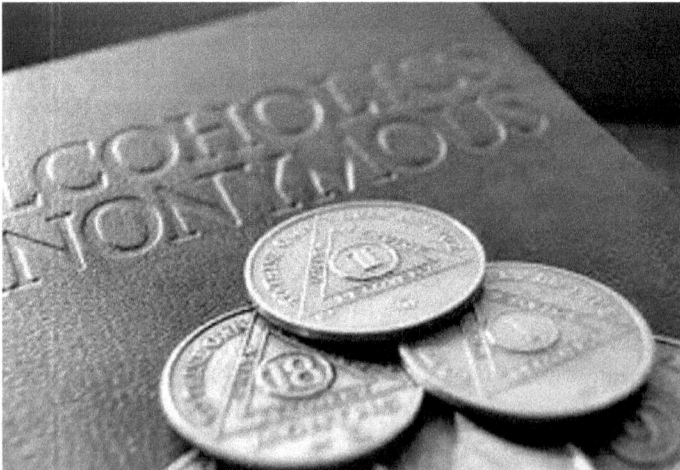

Taite Adams

Club Houses

If you're looking to have an image in AA, look around at the meetings you go to and take a look at who you're trying to impress.

This one can confuse the crap out of newcomers, and some uninitiated old-timers as well. Some AA meetings are held at what are referred to as "Clubhouses". These are centralized locations, that are not churches, schools, etc., and that generally have multiple meetings a day in the same location. The most important thing to note about Club Houses is that they are NOT AA Groups. In fact, they are required to be set up as separate businesses and each meeting that is held in the clubhouse then pays part of its collection to the Club House for the meeting space. There may also be several different types of meetings held in the location, such as AA, NA, Al-Anon, Coda, etc.

I am not "knocking" Club Houses at all. I got sober at one and my current Home Group is in an Alano Club. They have some tremendous benefits and just a few downsides. The benefits of Club Houses is that many are "open" all day long (some 24 hours) and until very late at night, regardless if there is a meeting going on or not. This provides a safe, recovery atmosphere for people to just go and "hang out" if they would like instead of sitting at home alone, staring at the clock and waiting for the next meeting to start. You can do that here instead. Many Club Houses also have very large memberships and do a lot of extra activities such as picnics, dances, pot lucks and marathon meetings on holidays such as Christmas, Thanksgiving and New Years.

The few downsides to Club Houses are that many people do mistake them for AA Groups. They are not. Authority, responsibility and accountability can get muddled. More so than at regular AA meetings, you may find people just hanging out at Club Houses who aren't necessarily looking to get sober as looking to stay off the street or stay out of trouble. Some may come to believe that simply hanging out a sober Club House is going to be enough to keep them sober. It most certainly will not. If you want to get sober and stay sober, there is still some other work to be done.

Kickstart Your Recovery

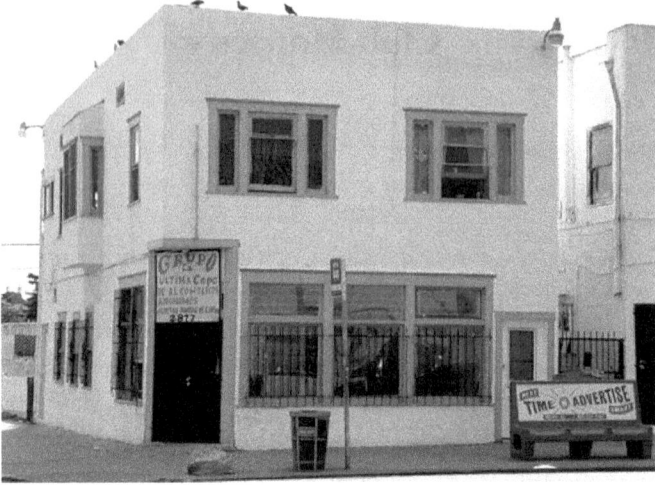

Taite Adams

If You Must ...Meetings Online and In Print

Why I go to meetings. "It is difficult to solve a problem with the same mind that created it."

Let me be clear up front on this, unless you are "house bound" or live outside the United States, this doesn't apply to you. And, even if you are either of the above, it likely doesn't apply to you. In AA's early years, there were very few Groups and meetings were few and far between. Some people traveled hours, or days, to get to an AA meeting only to wait weeks to attend their next meeting. And, guess what? They stayed sober!   Others, in remote parts of the world, were only able to communicate with other recovering alcoholics through written correspondence, again where they had to wait weeks or more for a reply. Guess what again? I'm not even going to say it.

Let's face it, we're spoiled. Today, there are over 2 million members of AA world-wide and over 115,000 AA Groups; and I think that these are conservative numbers.   In most cities and towns, there are meetings going on multiple times a day or just a short drive away. Yes, a majority of Groups are in the United States but this is a world-wide fellowship and the fact that you live in some small, remote country may not preclude your participation. You're all set Botswana - I just verified this. I have been in some serious 3rd world places, riding down the road only to look over and see that little blue AA sign hanging in a window somewhere. Comforting site, that.

However, if you live on Easter Island (they don't have meetings there, I checked), or are perhaps serving on a seagoing vessel for long periods of time, then Correspondence Meetings and Meetings Online may be for you.   There is a program called **Loners-Internationalists Meeting (LIM)**, that is a service available for situations such as this and is sponsored by AA World Services.   Go to (http://www.aa.org/en_pdfs/smf-123_en.pdf) for more information on this program.

Kickstart Your Recovery

If you would like to check out AA Meetings online, there are many. You can find a good directory of Online AA Meetings at (http://aa-intergroup.org/directory.php). However, let me state one more time that these should not be a substitute for live meetings if you can get to them. When the program of AA was founded, there was no internet and Live Meetings are real people sharing real issues in living color. A glaring characteristic of many alcoholics, recovering or not, is the search for an easier softer way. Are you looking for e-recovery or real recovery from alcoholism? It comes down to willingness, really. If you are in downtown Chicago, surrounded by AA meetings and can only be bothered to click a link on your laptop to attend a meeting, there's an issue there. If you, however, do live on Easter Island and would give your big toe to attend a real live meeting if one were there (hint: start one), getting online and doing what you can with what you have at the moment shows your complete willingness to work for your sobriety. Make sense?

Finally, if you have some physical limitations or are home bound for whatever reason, there is help. AA has what is called a "Special Needs" Committee that is comprised of members who want to help you get to meetings. What you need to do is Google "AA intergroup" and then your city or town. Give those guys a call and let them know your situation. They will put you in touch with your local Special Needs Committee and/or take your name and number and have someone get back to you who can give you some assistance in either getting you to an AA meeting or bringing an AA meeting to you.

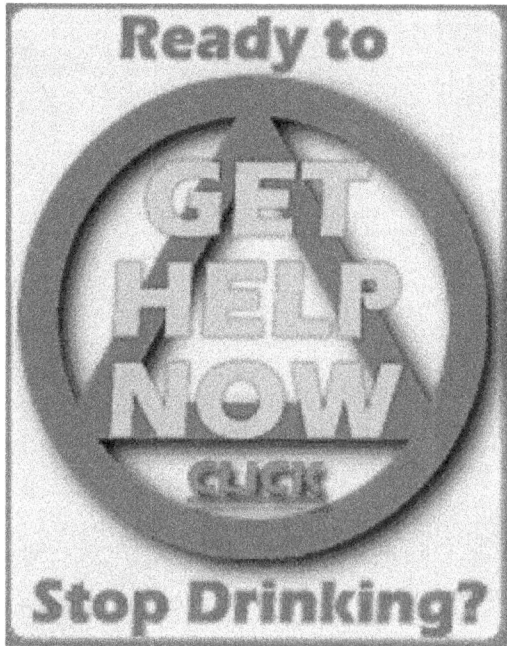

Taite Adams

What's Up With Those Slogans

The AA slogans are like railings for the Steps.

Step into any AA Group meeting room or AA Club House and you will likely see cards around the room or even framed posters on the walls with catchy little slogans. When your mind clears enough to take in what's said in the meetings, you'll also notice these phrases thrown out quite a bit. While even many oldtimers may think that some of these are a bit corny, there is no doubt that AA is chock full of slogans and that they do have their uses.

The slogans actually act as compact little reminders of the principles of the program that can be repeated, discussed or plastered on your wall to keep you on track. Many of these slogans may seem simple enough on the surface but, remember, simplicity does not always mean superficiality. So, before you scoff at the slogans and discount them completely, remember a few simple ideas. The slogans serve as inspiration to those participating in the program and also provide a sense of belonging and togetherness. Here are just a few of AAs main slogans and their meanings:

- **Let Go and Let God**. The advice here is to develop the capacity to let go of problems. It involves putting faith in a higher power in the belief that things will turn out as they should. The individual is not the master of the whole universe and by letting go they acknowledge this. If people try to control too much of their own life it will just mean that they are getting in the way.
- **One Day at a Time**. This is probably the most famous of all the AA slogans. It reminds the member that they have no control over tomorrow. Their only job is to do the best they can today. Attempting to fight tomorrow's battles tends to do a lot more harm than good. There is already enough that needs doing today.
- **This Too Shall Pass**. Life is constantly changing and so are the things that people will experience. Even if problems seem

huge at the time they are unlikely to seem so important in the future. This slogan is a reminder to people to hang in there with the knowledge that nothing lasts forever. It is similar to the idea that "time heals all wounds".

- **Think, Think, Think**. Acting rashly often leads to negative results. This catchphrase reminds people to think carefully before they do something they might later regret.

Very little in AA is "original" stuff and many of these catch phrases have been borrowed from the world's great spiritual traditions. There are literally hundreds of AA slogans and, while some may not make sense to you or just seem really stupid, there may be others that are of great benefit and do offer that additional inspiration that is needed in compact form at just the right moment.

"The slogans are Band-aids; The steps are the cure; your Higher Power is the doctor."

The 12 Steps - To What?

All we ask is that you completely change your attitude as soon as possible

As a newcomer in AA, or a treatment center resident, we'll hear such things as "the same person that walked through those doors will drink again" and "the only thing you have to change is - everything." Well, they're right. Getting sober and staying sober requires the changing of not only actions but of attitudes as well and that's a tough nut to crack without some sort of formula or process to follow. Enter the 12 Steps.

While attendance at meetings is a key part of recovery, as are other activities, at the heart of the program is the 12 Steps and you will be hard pressed to find a meeting room that doesn't have these prominently displayed for all to see. It is strongly suggested that you work the Steps with a Sponsor, someone who has experience with this and with some time in recovery. The main premise of beginning the 12 Steps is that we admit to using something outside ourselves to change the way we feel, and have used it to excess. There is that admission of powerlessness and unmanageability that, whether conscious or not, many of us made before finally asking for help.

What working the 12 Steps does is allow us to take a look at the role our ego and pride has played in our lives, particularly in our addictions and our actions. The personal reflection that takes place and confession actually helps to establish new levels of self awareness and helps to overcome the shame that nearly all of us have, whether we are initially aware of it or not. Scientists believe that this process may actually help to "rewire the brain" in that the pre-frontal cortex is reinvigorated. Our sense of self is impacted profoundly by the process of making amends, that also serves to alleviate feelings of guilt and limit stressors that could trigger relapse. Finally, and certainly not least, there is a renewed spiritual connection that takes place through this entire process. This is, of course, very difficult to measure but there is no doubt that this is an essential element to, and byproduct of, working the Steps.

Kickstart Your Recovery

Most alcoholics would rather die than learn anything about themselves. In fact, they do.

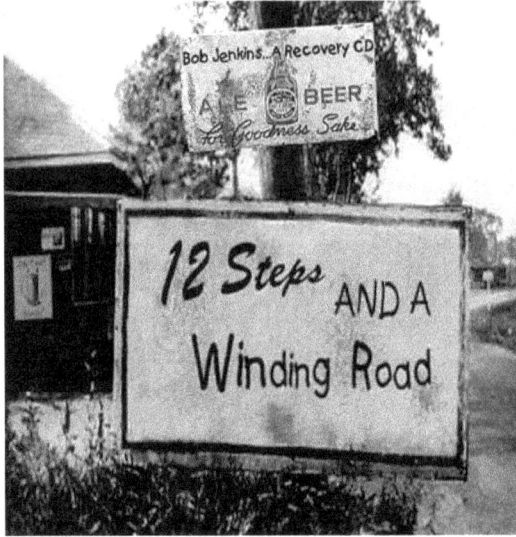

What is a Sponsor and Do I Need One?

"I would be fine, If I listened to opinions other than just my own......."

Many newcomers in AA look for "loopholes" and reasons why they shouldn't "have" to take suggestions. One very common suggestion is that you get a Sponsor. If you are looking for a loophole, here it is: there is no mention of sponsorship in the Big Book at all. In fact, in the earliest days of AA, the term sponsor was not in AA jargon. However, it wasn't too long before a few hospitals in both Akron, OH ("birthplace" of AA) and New York began accepting patients under the "alcoholic" diagnosis only if a sober member of AA would agree to "sponsor" that person. The sponsor would actually bring that person to the hospital, visit them, handle them at discharge and then bring them into the fold of AA once out. Through the early months of recovery, the sponsor would be there ready to listen and answer questions whenever needed. This practice has since become a long-standing custom and essential element of the AA Program of recovery. AA defines a sponsorship in this way: *"An alcoholic who has made some progress in the recovery program who shares that experience on a continuous, individual basis with another who is attempting to attain or maintain sobriety through A.A."*

This is another instance of recognizing that "my best thinking got me here" and that I need to learn how to ask for and accept help from someone else. I know a lot about getting drunk and screwing up my life but next to nothing about how to get and stay sober. One of the foundations of this program is that we help each other to succeed and Sponsorship is set up to do just that. So, do you need a sponsor? Well, only if you want to recover. But before you grab the first "sober" person you see at a meeting for the job, let's clarify just what a sponsor's role really is and some things that you may want to consider when selecting a sponsor.

Sponsoring yourself is like using unskilled labor.

Kickstart Your Recovery

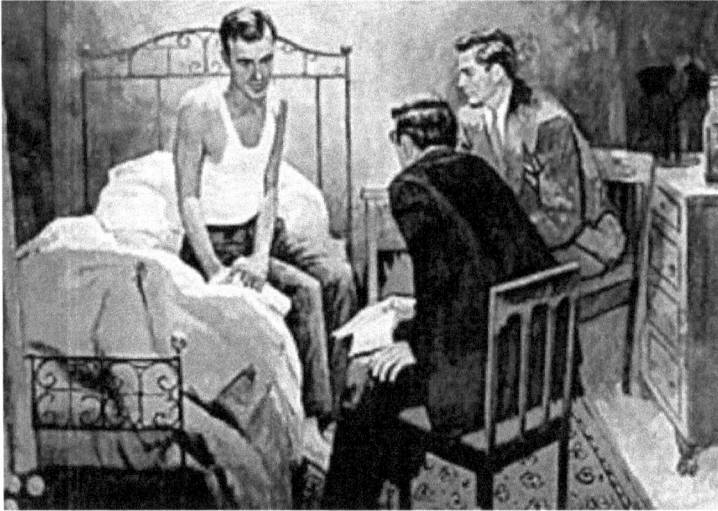

A Sponsor's Role

"S.P.O.N.S.O.R. = Sober Person Offering Newcomers Suggestions On Recovery."

There is little debate that the sponsor's key role is to act as guide through the 12 Steps. It is understood that the Steps are never to be worked alone and should be undertaken with the help and guidance of a sponsor. The methods through which a sponsor does this will be varied. Many do it with the Big Book as a guide and others with the "12 and 12". Some may use workbooks or other literature, or none at all. The time frame with which this is all carried out varies as well. A lot of sponsors will sponsor other people based on how they were "sponsored", and so on. There are no hard and fast rules to this.

A sponsor will generally, first and foremost, set out to get to know their new sponsee (that's you) a little bit more. They may do this by asking you to call them every day or meet them at a meeting. Asking you to do these things is also a gauge of your willingness to work a program. Another role that the sponsor plays is help you get acquainted with the fellowship and its meetings. This is someone who will answer questions, show you the ropes, and act as a general guide in learning to live a new way of life.

While a sponsor's primary role is to guide you through working the Steps, they are so much more and most certainly don't go away once that process is complete. They will often act as an emotional sounding board and point out things about yourself that you may not want to hear or that may be painful. These are all things that are necessary for growth. They will also share their own experiences with you about their disease, their recovery and their growth.

Many times, sponsorship leads to strong, life-time bonds never experienced before. Through the process of one alcoholic helping another, both are able to grow, learn and change. There are so many benefits of getting a sponsor, not the least of which is always having a person with whom you can share your thoughts and feelings about anything you wish. Some of the finest friendships have developed from this idea of sponsorship and most alcoholics, who are recovering, find a sponsor an important part of the process.

. . . what comes to us alone may be garbled by our own rationalization and wishful thinking. The benefit of talking to another person is that we can get his direct comment and counsel on our situation. . . . TWELVE STEPS AND TWELVE TRADITIONS, p. 60

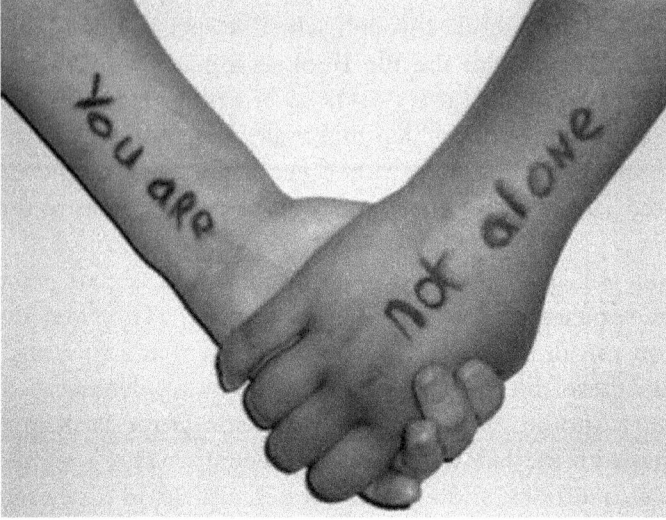

Choosing a Sponsor That's Right for You

"When the student is ready, the teacher will appear."

Many people in AA joke that choosing their first sponsor was like asking someone to be their Valentine. It's uncomfortable, awkward and many times, you're terrified of what will happen if they say "yes". Before we get to the actual asking part, there are some things that you want to consider in looking for a sponsor. Here are a few:

- A year or more of sobriety
- The same gender as you (there are exceptions to this rule)
- Emphasizes the Steps and Traditions of the Program
- Has what we want in terms of recovery and serenity

These are just some basic guidelines to use in your search. I could list a slew of them that would just serve to bog you down and ensure that you never find anyone to fit the bill. Remember, these are other "human beings", not saints. What we are looking for is someone who is successfully working the program of AA and is willing to help you do the same. If you get stuck here, don't be afraid to ask group members for help and suggestions. I've heard valid arguments that perhaps I'm not going to be the best judge of who is right for me when I first walk through the doors of AA. While not knowing that I was doing it at the time, I did have help finding my first sponsor and even asking her. I was that unsure, afraid and intimidated. I was also willing and got it done, though.

Before we wrap this up, let's be clear about what a sponsor is NOT. A sponsor is not a bank, a landlord, a boss, or a relative. They don't lend money, provide housing, give you a job, or have any blood relation to you whatsoever. These things muddy the waters and take away from the true purpose of the relationship. A sponsor is also not a therapist and should never do anything to exploit their sponsee in any way, shape or form. Yes, advice on recovery and living sober may be dispensed but this is done through the context of the sponsor's own experiences in recovery, not as an expert in psychiatry or as a psychologist. Also, it is not the sponsee's role to wash cars, weed gardens or act as a chauffeur for anyone in the name of sobriety. A sponsor has a sacred and abiding trust towards their sponsees. Morally and ethically a sponsor may not take advantage of this relationship bond in any way, at any time.

That being said, sponsorship is a vital part of the program of Alcoholics Anonymous and it is strongly suggested that you jump in and start your journey with a guide. As far as just How to ask another member to Sponsor you, simply start going to lots of meetings (90 in 90 is good) and watch the members that are sharing. Focus on those that seem to be happy, content and have something that you want. Chances are, they will make a good sponsor. Approach that person either before or after a meeting, introduce yourself and ask them if they would be willing to be your sponsor. If they say no, it's not a reflection on you at all. There may be a hundred reasons for this. Don't dwell on it - just look for someone else who's recovery inspires you.

...we will be victorious if we have not forgotten how to learn. -Rosa Luxemburg

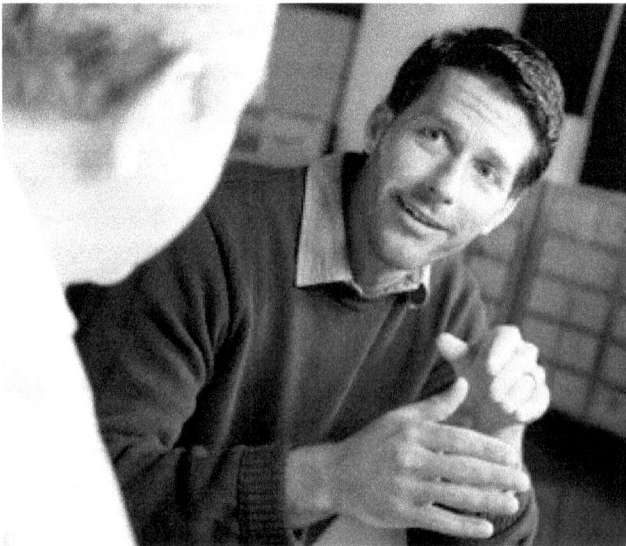

The God Factor

"First of all, we had to quit playing God. It didn't work." — *Alcoholics Anonymous*

If God is your co-pilot, SWITCH SEATS!!!

It is sometimes declared that Alcoholics Anonymous is a religious movement. The basis for these claims usually stems from the focus on a higher power in the 12 Steps. In reality, it is not "religious" in nature at all, rather it is spiritual as members are able to form their own conception of a higher power as they see fit. The crux of the recovery program, once again, is the essence of learning to rely on a higher power and coming to realize that "I'm not it".

AA did get its initial influence from a Christian evangelical group, known as the Oxford Group. The spiritual philosophy of the Oxford Group involved:

- Belief in God
- Regular and rigorous self-examination in order to monitor character flaws
- Making amends for any wrongdoing
- Admitting one's faults to at least one other person

These same principles were incorporated into AAs 12 Steps of recovery, except that AA adopts the concept of an all-inclusive "Higher Power" as opposed to mandating that everyone believe in God. This ensures that everyone can make a beginning here. Here is a bit more about how that works.

We needed to ask ourselves but one short question. "Do I now believe, or am I even willing to believe, that there is a Power greater than myself?" As soon as a man can say that he does believe, or is willing to believe, we emphatically assure him that he is on his way. ALCOHOLICS ANONYMOUS, p. 47

There is a higher power.

I'm not it.

The Higher Power Concept - But I'm Jewish, an Atheist, an Agnostic, Buddhist, a Wiccan...

Every now and again take a good look at something not made with hands - a mountain, a star, the turn of a stream. There will come to you wisdom and patience and solace and, above all, the assurance that you are not alone in the world. -Sidney Lovett

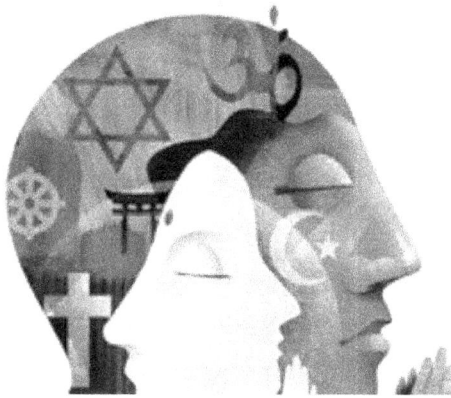

The thing that is needed to begin recovery is some sort of belief in a higher power, something outside of myself that is in charge. I know that I tried everything under my own power for a good long time to either stop or control my drinking and using. I just couldn't do it. There is no requirement in AA that one believes in God or in any specific conception of a Higher Power. Yes, there are mentions of "God" in the literature and even some Christian-based prayers that are said in the meetings. These aren't designed to trick you into converting to anything. A lot of this is born from Tradition and the roots of the program (good luck trying to change any of that).

Regardless, if you are Jewish, Catholic, Baptist, Atheist, or anything under the sun, there is no belief or "non-belief" system that AA has not been able to accommodate over the years. Atheists can use the power of the group (**G**roup **O**f **D**runks) as their higher power, others use **G**ood **O**rderly **D**irection, and still others use the impersonal force of nature. The only guiding principle is that the "higher power" must be a power greater than yourself, which all of these would certainly be.

While the Group of Drunks does work for many, AA does ask that members be willing to keep the door open to the possibility of a higher power that is spiritual in nature. This also does not dictate that members conform their beliefs to any particular God or religion. In fact, I've read a few things attributed to Bill W that said something along the lines of how glad he was when religious leaders from varied traditions found the Twelve Steps to be compatible with their religion. The concepts are ancient, and they existed before Christ. It is also quite common for this "belief" to develop and evolve over time, particularly as a result and byproduct of working the 12 Steps.

Yes, belief in a Higher Power can make life easier. I know that it goes against our very nature as alcoholics to want to give up any sort of control. Here is a list of benefits to consider in doing so:

- People who are attempting to escape a life of addiction can feel overwhelmed by that task and may have found that they don't have the ability to defeat their problem alone. In the AA program they can rely on a power greater than themselves to give them the strength they need.

- When people believe in a higher power they will usually find it easier to forgive other people who have wronged them. (ie - letting go of resentments)

- The individual will need to face many challenges in recovery. It can be a great source of comfort to believe in a higher power that is providing them with help.

- In AA, they encourage members to learn how to let go. This means adopting a completely new approach to life. When people develop the ability to let go with the help of a higher power it brings them peace of mind and contentment.

- Belief in a higher power can give people a sense of purpose in their life. This new approach to life can strengthen their recovery and reduce the risk of relapse. Those who follow a spiritual path claim that it brings a great deal of happiness to their life.

- All spiritual paths encourage the individual to develop as humans. This will usually mean that they become more loving and mentally healthy. Addicts tend to be self-absorbed, but belief in a higher power can help to combat this tendency.

Again, this wasn't an overwhelming issue for me when I "joined" AA and committed to getting sober. I knew that my being "in charge" provided disastrous results and it was actually a relief to give up control, finally, in both the area of my addictions and in other matters in my life. This is an evolutionary process for most and my belief system has grown, evolved and enriched so much over the years. All it took in the beginning, however, was an ounce of willingness and I certainly had that.

My friend suggested what then seemed a novel idea. . . .
"Why don't you choose your own conception of God?" That statement hit me hard. It melted the icy intellectual mountain in whose shadow I had lived and shivered many years I stood in the sunlight at last. It was only a matter of being willing to believe in a Power greater than myself. Nothing more was required of me to make my beginning. ALCOHOLICS ANONYMOUS, p. 12

Kickstart Your Recovery

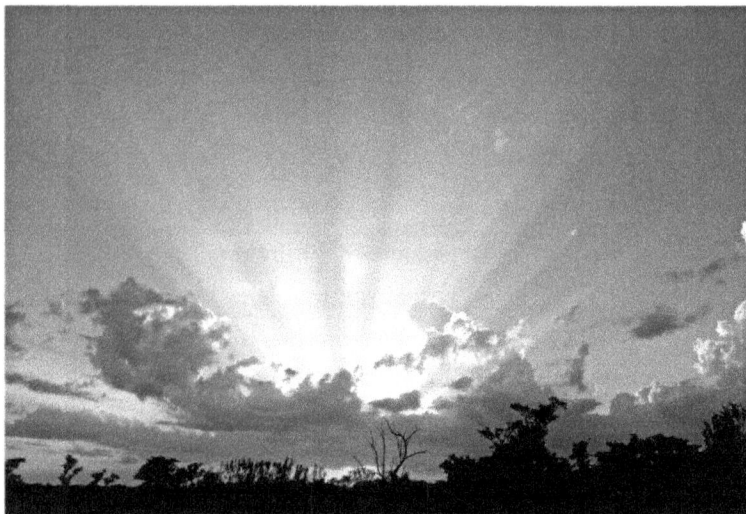

Families and Relationships

"The primary fact that we fail to recognize is our total inability to form a true partnership with another human being." - Twelve Steps and Twelve Traditions, p. 53

No one comes into AA or recovery on a high note in their lives and a lot of times that means that there is some sort of family turmoil going on in the background, or in the forefront of their everyday living. There are a few things that I know for sure. One is that most people do not understand the disease of alcoholism at all. Heck, I have it and didn't understand anything about it for years. That being said, it's a lot to ask other people to just completely change their opinions of you simply because you've managed to stay away from a drink for a few days, weeks or months. Everything takes time (you'll hear this a lot in AA). Another thing I know is that everything changes. I've learned both through my personal experiences and through observing the experiences of others that things simply work out the way they are supposed to if the alcoholic stays sober and keeps doing the right thing. Sometimes that's easier said than done, I know.

"TIME = Things I Must Earn"

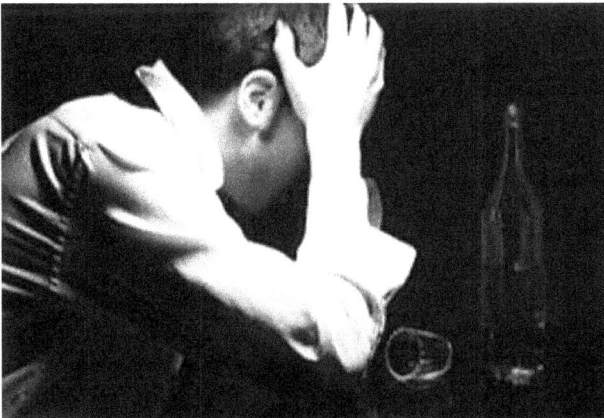

My Spouse Left Me, Won't Speak to Me, Won't Leave Me Alone...

It is the great obsession of every Al-Anon, that some day he or she will learn to control and enjoy their drinker

There's a chapter in the Big Book that is quite dated and a bit controversial, called "To Wives". Bill W (one of AAs founders) wrote this chapter to the strong objection of many, including his wife Lois, who actually would have preferred being asked to write the section. The Chapter, unfortunately, turned out to be a blueprint for how a wife should act around her newly recovering alcoholic husband, or rather how her husband would want her to act. Perhaps you can see why these ideas and, possibly some of the verbiage, would be a bit dated. There is plenty of wisdom in AA and most treatment centers, however to help you deal with these issues prudently.

Being in a relationship while trying to get sober is never easy, even if your significant other is your #1 cheerleader and biggest supporter. The reason for this is that recovery takes a tremendous amount of commitment, dedication and brings forth a great deal of change - both for the alcoholic and everyone who comes into contact with them. Unfortunately, when we begin to get serious about our recovery, we can start appearing distant from our families, especially our spouse. What happens in a recovery program, in AA Groups and with a sponsor can be difficult to explain and these changes that are occurring can't always be laid out for someone else in black and white. That can be very frustrating for family members that want to support us and stay involved and also for the alcoholic who wants to fight to maintain those strong bonds.

What is most important to remember is this. Recovery must come first. If you don't stay sober, at some point, these family members, spouses, children, significant others and bonds that you are trying to maintain are going to disappear anyway. This is something that I struggled with for years. I was told over and over again that "anything you put before your recovery, you're going to lose." I simply didn't believe it, until one thing after another continued to slip away and, finally, I lost my 3 year old child. That was the breaking point for me. I had gotten to a place where I knew that I had to recover first and then those relationships would be there if they were meant to be - and they definitely were.

If you do have family members, a spouse, children or significant other who very much want to be involved in your recovery, that's fantastic. What you may want to do is refer them to one of the family groups, such as Al-Anon or Alateen, so that they are also able to have a recovery program and people to talk to. When they say that alcoholism is a "family disease", they are not only referring to the genetic nature of passing this on through generations. When there is an active alcoholic in the family, in some way, shape or form, everyone suffers. People blame, take on more than their share, become angry, depressed and so on. We all deserve to recover and the family groups understand and can help with this.

"Years of living with an alcoholic is almost sure to make any wife or child neurotic. The entire family is, to some extent, ill." ALCOHOLICS ANONYMOUS, p. 122

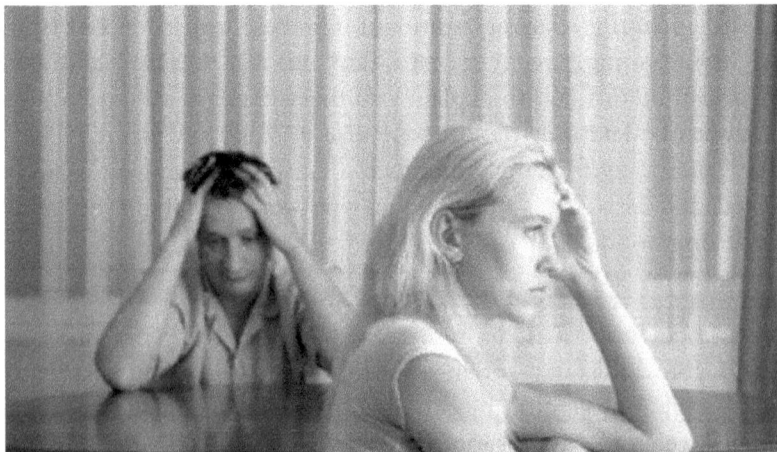

Taite Adams

No One Trusts Me

"When your prospect has made such reparation as he can to his family, and has thoroughly explained to them the new principles by which he is living, he should proceed to put those principles into action at home." AA, 2001, p. 98

Well, why should they really? One of the saddest elements of addiction is that those closest to the alcoholic or addict are the ones that get hurt the most, over and over again. Loved ones try to control the impossible, they try to stop caring, or finally they just detach with love if they are able. We leave in our wake a mountain of lies, broken promises, financial ruin and shame. Re-gaining any sort of trust is not easy and certainly will not happen overnight. Here is what you need to do to get started with rebuilding any sort of trust:

- Stop using drugs and alcohol
- Change your lifestyle
- Change "who" you are by becoming painstakingly honest and backing up your words with action.
- Time. How much time? As long as it takes.

Trust takes a lot longer to rebuild than it does to destroy. Family members who are trying to rebuild trust with a recovering addict are not starting out on an even playing field, as you would with someone you just met. They are trying to climb out of a deep well of hurt, disappointment, and fear. Family members also need to commit to being honest about their feelings and expectations.

One thing to remember is that Trust is not the same thing as love and forgiveness. Our loved ones can love us and forgive us but still not trust us again yet. Love and forgiveness are choices. Trust is also a choice but takes honesty and time. The key is for the recovering alcoholic to begin to build on small victories, become more predictable in their actions, have their actions match their words, and continue to be completely honest under all circumstances. These elements, a commitment to communication, and time are keys to rebuilding trust when one or both of you are recovering.

It took me many years to rebuild trust with family members. I still had loving relationships with them and still spent time with them. However, I had done a lot of damage and had been so dishonest with them for so long that it was understandable for them not to give me back that trust right away. I had to continue to do trustworthy things and back up my words with appropriate and positive actions. The fact that the trust took a long time to come back, makes it all the more cherished and something that I would never want to break again.

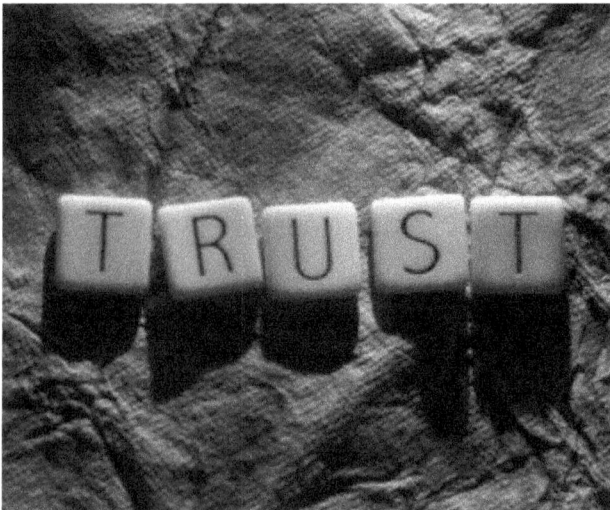

The Job, Work, Career

If drinking is interfering with your work, you're probably a heavy drinker. If work is interfering with your drinking, you're probably an alcoholic.

Many people, myself included, who enter rehab or seek to get sober are worried about the state of their jobs or careers. In a lot of cases, these were in jeopardy well before making the choice to get some help. Countless missed days from work, poor work product or performance, and crummy attitudes are just a few of the "clues" that we tend to give off that something is amiss. I generally quit jobs just before I was about to be fired so that I could continue to claim that I had "never been fired". The few times that I did ask for help, I wasn't entirely honest about where I was going or for what purpose and the results were dismal. While many of us thought that we managed to hide our little problem quite well, don't be shocked if your employer has been in on the secret for quite some time and has even been at odds with just what to do about you.

Despite all of this, there are still fears and they are understandable. It is estimated that more than 25 percent of individuals struggling with addictions believe that they would experience negative job consequences if they sought treatment. People may fear losing a professional license, failing to get a promotion, losing authority or respect of subordinates, or also of losing the respect of supervisors and co-workers. In this current economy, it's understandable to fear losing one's job and being unable to find another one. However, times have changed a lot in recent years as more information becomes available about this disease and about recovery.

Employers are beginning to recognize the high cost of substance abuse in the workplace. The Bureau of National Affairs has reported that chemical dependency alone costs American businesses approximately $200 billion annually. Many employers are now providing addiction treatment through health insurance, as a company benefit, and through Employee Assistance Programs (EAPs). Some are even paying employees and providing other incentives to get treatment. When interviewing individuals who are in recovery, many who were employed at the time of treatment told their employer why they needed time off. Of those that told their employer they were going to attend drug rehab, a great many kept their job. There are exceptions, particularly if you have a job that involves handling controlled substances (such as nurses or doctors), or are responsible for public safety (such as airline pilots). In the end it all comes down to, once again, the fact that recovery has to come first. There is still plenty of hope, however, for getting the help you need and keeping your career intact if it is meant to be.

We feel that elimination of our drinking is but a beginning. A much more important demonstration of our principles lies before us in our respective homes, occupations and affairs. ALCOHOLICS ANONYMOUS, p. 19

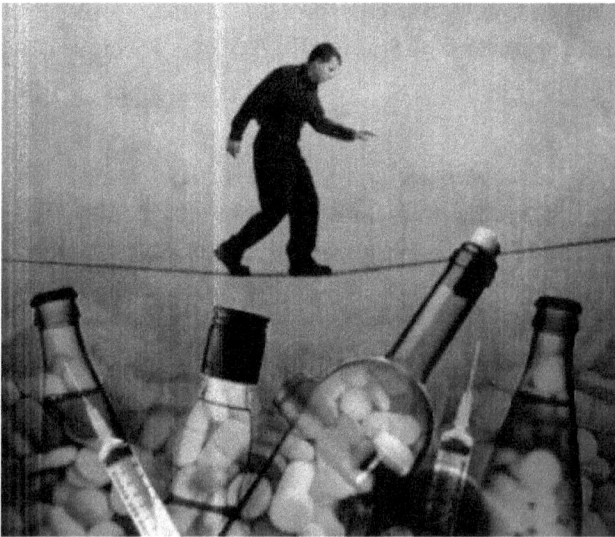

Making Career Changes - or Not

AA and recovery are full of paradoxes. You'll get told not to make any major changes for the first year and then, in the same breath, someone will say "the only thing that you need to change is - everything!". Well, they're both right in a sense. The first statement applies to your jumping into new relationships, making a major geographic move if you don't have to and other major life changes that may also include job and career. The second statement refers to the changes in our attitudes and belief systems that occur when we work a recovery program. This refers to a complete change in our outlook and how we see things. When it comes to making the choice get help, enter treatment, go to detox, or just start going to AA, job and career can certainly be affected. Career provides structure to many and loss of that, in the wake of trying to get sober, can be tough.

Statistics, and experience, show that alcoholics are above-average earners and quite high functioning in society, even in their addictions. In 2008, among the nearly 73 million binge and heavy alcohol users, nearly 80 percent had either full-time or part-time jobs, according to the Substance Abuse and Mental Health Services Administration, known as SAMHSA. And among the 17.8 million illicit drug users, 73 percent were employed. While the ego wishes to pat ourselves on the back for this, that isn't why I mention it. The fact is, with employment numbers like this, there is SO MUCH help available that it's a shame not to take advantage of it.

Remember that addiction is a disease, much like high blood pressure or diabetes. If you need hospitalization for diabetes, most employers would understand. Ideally, the same should hold true for addiction. You may also want to consider whether your time off for treatment would be covered under the Family and Medical Leave Act (FMLA). According to the Unites States Department of Labor, FMLA "entitles eligible employees of covered employers to take unpaid, job-protected leave for specified family and medical reasons with continuation of group health insurance coverage under the same terms and conditions as if the employee had not taken leave."

Not all jobs are protected by FMLA regulations, but many are, particularly in larger companies and if you have worked for your employer for some time. Information regarding FMLA can be found on the internet or by contacting your employer's human resources department. If you do not believe your employer will be receptive to your need for drug rehab or if FMLA is not an option, you can request time off for personal reasons. Also check out your companies EAP (Employee Assistance Program) for options.

If you do have to leave your job to get help, you may just be heading off the inevitable anyway. Like I said, I left several jobs, including my last one, just before the axe fell - even once writing a letter of resignation from a jail cell because I knew I wouldn't be making it to work the next day. If a job is "lost" in the quest for recovery, so be it. The opportunity to focus on your sobriety and to find a new job may be a blessing in disguise.

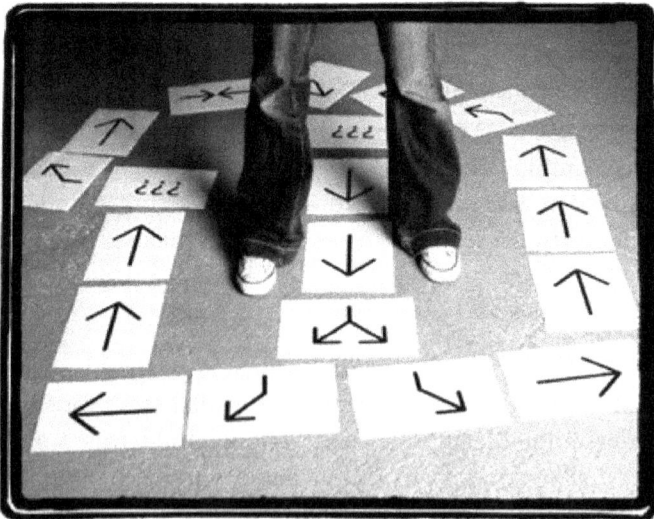

Taite Adams

What is a "Recovery Job"?

Never turn down a job because you think it's too small; you don't know where it can lead. -Julia Morgan

When I was getting ready to leave treatment this last time, I felt renewed, full of life and very fragile. I had finally "gotten it" after several years of resistance and did not want to do anything to screw it up. I was told that I needed to put my recovery first and that seemed easy enough because the rest of my life was a decent sized mess. I was faced, however, with the prospect of leaving treatment, finding a place to live, and seeking employment. This required a bit of soul searching and a lot of discussion because I was used to working in some higher-paying, stressful environments and did not feel like I was equipped just yet to return to one of these dens of iniquity. It was suggested that I get a "recovery job".

A "Recovery Job" is a simpler job than something that you are perhaps used to. It is a job that is low stress and probably much lower paying. Hours worked will vary but there is nothing wrong with an 8 hour work day that keeps you busy; it's the stress level and responsibility factor that we are concerned about here. The logic here is that there is enough for you to worry about early in sobriety without adding additional work and career stresses to the mix if you don't have to. In fact, the simpler you can make your life in all other areas, the better.

In my case, I went from high finance to file clerk. One thing I had to do was "dumb down" my resume a little bit so that I was not seen as being "overqualified" for everything. I had to take the Master's Degree and several recent jobs off of my resume. I started just a few days out of rehab with a temporary agency as a file clerk. I can tell you that the position was pretty low stress for me and I was pretty darn good at it. So good, in fact, that I was hired as a full-time permanent employee of that company. This led to other internal promotions over the course of several years and, after some time, I was working for the President and came clean about my background and my recovery. I continued to do well there until the company went out of business and I started my own business at 6 years sober.

Things happened for me just as they were supposed to. There are many more stories like this but sometimes it can be difficult to know just where to start when beginning in recovery with no job. Once in recovery, rejoining the mainstream of life can be challenging. Below are a few organizations that help people in recovery re-enter the workplace.

- America in Recovery (americainrecovery.org)
  America in Recovery is a non-profit effort to promote the hiring of people in recovery from alcohol and drug abuse as well as people with felony convictions. This no-charge hiring web site links job seekers and employers directly with each other.

- Community Voice Mail (CVM) (cvm.org)
  Provides free, personalized 24-hour voice mail access nationwide in order to empower people in crisis and transition by providing a direct link to jobs, housing and stability. CVM centers are listed by state on their web site.

- National H.I.R.E. Network (hirenetwork.org/workforce-professionals)
  The National H.I.R.E. Network (Helping Individuals with criminal records Re-Enter through Employment) serves as an information clearinghouse and provides leadership on public policy to promote the employment of people with criminal records. Under Resources and Assistance, there are listings by state of government agencies and community-based organizations that assist people with criminal records. These agencies and organizations can be of assistance in providing job-related and legal services, answering questions arising from having a criminal record, or offering referrals to other useful organizations.

Sponsee: "When will I get a good job?"
Sponsor: "When you are ready."

Taite Adams

Sponsee: "How will I know I am ready?"
Sponsor: "You'll have a good job."

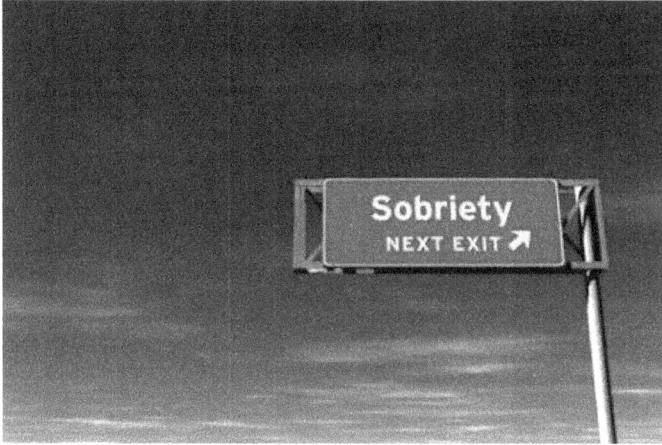

Got Consequences?

"It all works out in the end...if it hasn't worked out yet, it's not the end."

How many times have we said, or heard another alcoholic or addict say, "I'm not hurting anybody. I'm only hurting myself."? Nothing could be further from the truth. For over 30 years now, the U.S. has been fighting its "War on Drugs", yet we have seen an increase in crime, increase in healthcare costs, and an alarming increase in the use of dangerous substances. The fact is that the effects of addiction are far reaching and can be seen in the home, on the job, in churches, and in schools. I can guarantee you than not one single person comes into a recovery program without some sort of consequences from their disease. They are a prerequisite to sobriety. Whether you have a DUI, strained marriage, job loss, bankruptcy, loss of liver function or just an overwhelming feeling of fear and uselessness, it counts.

Everyone entering recovery has consequences stemming from their disease. It's one of the ties that binds us together so strongly. A benefit of meetings and sharing with others is that you will always find someone who has been through the same circumstances that you are currently in, that can share their sober experiences with you, and give you hope that everything will be ok and work out as it should. In recovery, we understand our triggers, the rituals and the patterns that accompany our various self-destructive behaviors; we can be a witness to all of it. But it is not until we place a value on the consequences of our behavior - a value that is greater than the motivation for that behavior -- that we are motivated to make a change. Until then, we'll just continue to build up a big steaming pile of consequences that will get infinitely worse as time, and our disease, progresses.

"When the door of happiness closes, another opens, but often times we look so long at the closed door, that we don't see the one which has been opened for us."

Kickstart Your Recovery

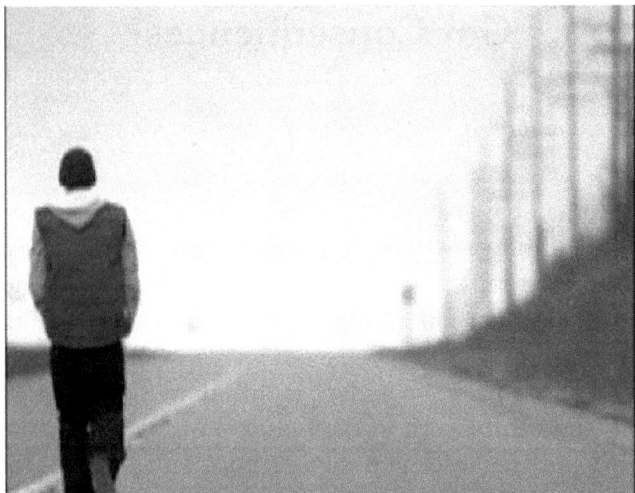

Health, Family, Legal, Financial

However confused the scene of our life appears, however torn we may be who now do face that scene, it can be faced, and we can go on to be whole. -Muriel Rukeyser

The impact of addiction can be far-reaching. Many of us had no idea how many areas of our lives were being affected by our alcohol and drug use, or simply had no desire to take a good hard look at it. In fact, consequences were being racked up in good measure in our health, family relationships, our dealings with society, and our financial affairs. Not so sure about this? Consider these ideas:

- **Health** - If left unchecked, the substance is always going to win. Alcoholism and addiction is a disease of the brain, and drugs change brain chemistry, which results in a change in behavior. Aside from the obvious behavioral consequences of addiction, the negative effects on a person's health are potentially devastating. While addicts use drugs to "feel better," the unintended consequences include, but are not limited to, overdose, HIV/AIDS, stroke, cardiovascular disease, and a host of related maladies.
- **Family** - One of the saddest aspects of the insidious nature of drug addiction is that by the time an addict realizes they have a problem, that problem has already taken a heavy toll on the family. Parents in treatment centers tell counselors and therapists that they want to "get their kids back," as drug addiction has taken over to the point where the courts have been forced to remove the children from the home. Husbands and wives, brothers and sisters, and sadly children are all impacted. Families can be sources of strength and support, or they can passively enable the addiction to advance. Families can share in the victory over drug addiction, or they can be the victims of it.
- **Legal** - The news media reports daily struggles with theft, drive-by shootings, drug busts, illegal trafficking and manufacturing of drugs, and arrests for crimes ranging from child neglect to murder. Look closer and chances are great that you will uncover a drug addiction component to any of these

stories. This is just the "big picture". Our "personal picture" usually isn't very pretty either. It often includes such things as multiple DUIs, probation violations, drug arrests, family court battles, civil suits and so on. The stress of the potential losses here can be overwhelming.

- **Financial** - Beyond the personal health issues, beyond the devastating effect on families, beyond community crime statistics, drug addiction has a major impact on the American economy. The National Institute on Drug Abuse (NIDA) reported that some $67 billion per year is the impact that drug addiction has on this country. This total includes the cost of law enforcement, incarceration, treatments, traffic injuries, lost time in the workplace, etc. Drug addiction causes impaired reasoning, and therefore the crime rate is dramatically impacted by drug use. Addicts have a much higher likelihood of committing crimes than others. Again, this is "big picture" stuff. Many of us, on the personal level are looking a losing homes, cars, jobs and paying legal fees that we can't afford. Again, major stressors.

It takes a lot of courage to face the consequences our actions have caused and, in many cases, to be able to even recognize them in the first place. If you go to treatment or AA, you will be in an environment where you will get the support that you need to face these consequences head on and hear the experiences of others who have successfully traveled this road before you. That was a huge benefit for me. When I got sober, I had a shit-pile of consequences. I was broke, had no place to live, no job, was in some serious legal trouble, and was losing custody of my child. I had a lot on my plate and got all the help I needed to deal with it. Things worked out just fine for me in all areas, because I stayed sober and kept putting my recovery first.

There is no such thing as a problem without a gift for you in its hands. -Richard Bach

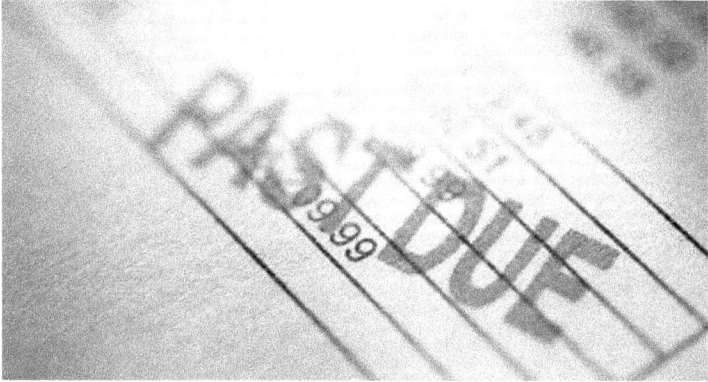

Old Friends and Stomping Grounds

"I didn't want to go to A.A. I had lost a lot of friends to A.A.!"

"Sometimes the hardest decision in life is which bridge to cross and which one to burn"

The thought of having to stay away from old drinking buddies and potential situations that may act as triggers for a relapse is enough to create boatloads of stress and defiance in many alcoholic's minds. I wasn't too worried about either because I didn't have many friends left and wasn't "going out" anymore at the end. I was, however, concerned about never being able to enjoy the bar scene again and projecting forward to holidays where I wouldn't be able to just have a beer or a glass of wine to celebrate. Note: I never just had A beer or A glass of wine with anything - ever. One unexpected benefit of recovery is that you pretty quickly learn who your real friends are, and aren't. I had several people make the drive to visit me in rehab that I would have never expected to reach out. There are others that I never heard from again.

When we get sober, many of these former "drinking buddies" are, unfortunately, toxic to our recovery. They may not understand the disease of addiction and don't know how to stop enabling. If they also have a problem with substance abuse, chances are that is going to take priority over any friendship with you and they certainly don't want your recovery acting as a mirror that's showing them the reality of their lives. Some may have tried to quit unsuccessfully and will be disheartened to see someone else recovering. Even if they don't have a problem, they may wish to enjoy alcohol socially without worrying about their influence on your recovery.

How do you know if a relationship is toxic to your recovery? Pseudo-friends and even some family members may discourage you from getting help. They'll tell you that you don't really have a drug or alcohol problem, recovery is a waste of time, or that relapse is inevitable. They may try bullying you to party with them, or use drugs in front of you.

Others may employ more subtle tactics, such as using your past behavior as leverage against you, holding onto resentments, making it difficult for you to get to meetings or therapy appointments, or belittling your efforts to get well. Even non-drinking buddies can be enablers. When family members refuse to work on their own issues, they may stay stuck in old patterns of minimizing, rescuing and enabling without realizing that they are sabotaging the person they most want to help.

Addicts with toxic relationships must be proactive in taking steps to safeguard their recovery. There is a general rule in recovery to stay away from the people, places and things associated with past drug and alcohol use. Maintaining relationships with people who drink or use is strongly associated with relapse. Early in recovery, it can be difficult to separate the supportive relationships from the malicious motives of would-be saboteurs, which is why it is always important to talk through your concerns with a sponsor. Cutting ties with old friends who continue to use and people who are not supportive of your sobriety is one of the hardest parts of early recovery. These difficult decisions need to be made swiftly. Parting with your social circle can be devastating but it is an important part of creating a new life and, ultimately, brings a great sense of relief when you find that you are surrounded by people who truly care.

This isn't all doom and gloom. Not all relationships have to end. You can re-connect with the people that you have probably alienated during active addiction who were "quality friends". Family members, and sometimes friends, are willing to join you in your recovery process by learning more about the disease of addiction and attending Al-Anon meetings. Early recovery is also a time for making new friends and building a healthy support network. Positive friends, which can include people you meet at work, in school, in AA, doing sober activities will not only help you to avoid drinking but will build that enthusiasm for a more balanced life.

"We have good news and bad news here. The good news is you never have to drink again even if you want to. The bad news is that we're your new friends."

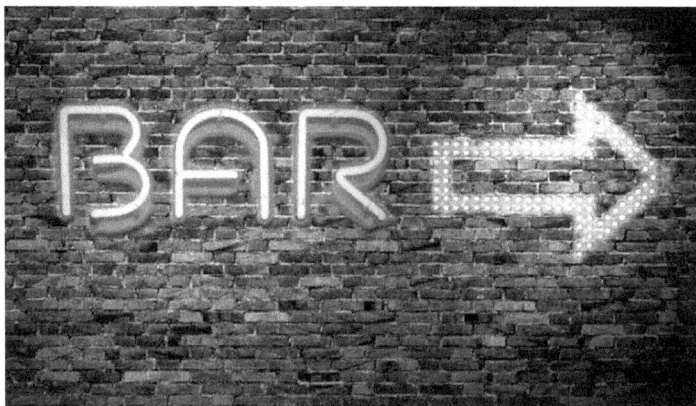

Taite Adams

Everyday Stuff in Sobriety

"...the greater part of our happiness or misery depends on our dispositions and not on our circumstances." -Martha Washington

Learning to do just about anything sober, including eating, sleeping and breathing, can be a task in itself. What a solid recovery program will teach us is how to handle these basic things, first and foremost, and then how to deal with every aspect of living life - sober. This includes the highs and the lows, the joys and the sorrows, through the gains and the losses. There is something called "emotional sobriety" that can be attained through working a program that will allow you to face any problem or circumstances and do it without picking up a drink or a drug. Alcoholics are notorious for celebrating victories as much as we are for drowning our sorrows so this is about balance. We have to learn to celebrate life, handle defeat and just "be" - sober. Some call this "Living Life on Life's Terms". Sounds trite to many but it's concise and relays the idea of what we are out to accomplish.

The idea of "twenty-four-hour living" applies primarily to the emotional life of the individual. Emotionally speaking, we must not live in yesterday, nor in tomorrow. AS BILL SEES IT, p. 284

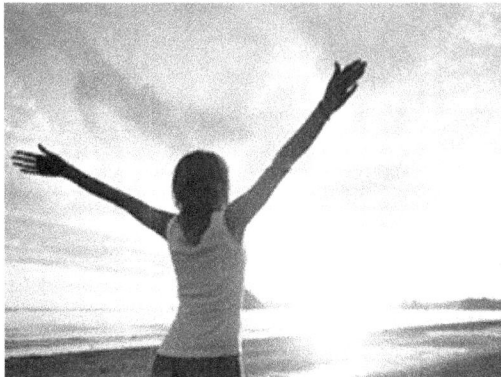

~ 99 ~

Taite Adams

Life on Life's Terms

Life is not always what one wants it to be, but to make the best of it as it is, is the only way of being happy. -Jennie Jerome Churchill

The idea of recovery is really to learn to how to incorporate positive principles and behaviors into one's lifestyle, so that when a real life situation arises, we are able to handle it without the use of a drink or a drug and, ideally, with some level of dignity and grace. We learn and practice these "principles" on all of our affairs, great and small, so that when major things do arise, we are able to summon those sober life experiences to deal with them. Living "life on life's terms" means just that, dealing with the ups and downs of life on a daily basis and doing it sober.

Most "normal" people are able to deal with normal life stuff without picking up a drink or being messed up. I never could. I couldn't imagine having to go to work, to school, or out to dinner without something in my system. If there was any sort of a life "curve ball", my first instinct was to turn up the volume on whatever it was I was already abusing. In reality, I was fearful of life and just wanted everything to go my way, all the time. I'd drown my sorrows when it didn't and celebrate when it did. This became exhausting, for me and everyone in my path. Real life doesn't work this way.

Being sober, I learned early on (Day 1), that I am no longer in charge. In fact, I never was but I just had to realize this. I also learned that most of the things that happen in life are beyond my scope of control. This didn't piss me off at all. It was a great revelation, in fact. I felt finally free to let go and stop trying to control everyone and everything in my path. Life on life's terms took on new meaning for me and I was able to start seeing things that were happening in life for what they were. They were just occurrences or situations and I could choose to accept them as they were or not. I read this very early in my sobriety and even had it laminated because, to me, it was so profound:

"And acceptance is the answer to all *of my problems today. When I am disturbed it is because I find some person, place, thing, or situation — some fact of my life — unacceptable to me, and I can find no serenity until I accept that person, place, thing, or situation as being exactly the way it is supposed to be at this moment. ..*

...Unless I accept life completely on life's terms, I cannot be happy. I need to concentrate not so much on what needs to be changed in the world as what needs to be changed in me and in my attitudes." -Alcoholics Anonymous Pg 417

Old adages ring true, "Most folks really are about as happy as they make their minds up to be." Perhaps you've faced some horrible injustice. You have every right to be angry and to express your needs and feelings. You also have the right to heal, to adjust (change), to overcome, and to transform. Simple choice: stay stuck or grow.

Everything has its wonders, even darkness and silence, and I learn, whatever state I may be in, therein to be content. -Helen Keller

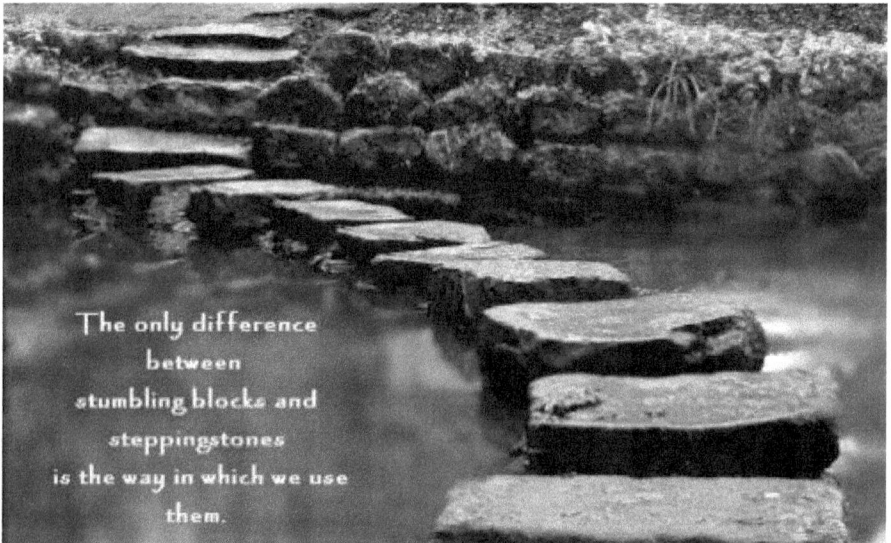

The only difference between stumbling blocks and steppingstones is the way in which we use them.

H.A.L.T.

"The good news is you get your emotions back. The bad news is you get your emotions back."

An important part of getting sober is learning how to take care of ourselves and listen to "clues" our bodies and minds give us that things may not be quite right. A popular acronym used in AA is H.A.L.T., which stands for "don't get too Hungry, Angry, Lonely, or Tired." If you do, you should obviously stop (halt) and address these things as they have a tendency to create confused or muddled feelings like depression and anxiety that may lead to a relapse if left unchecked for a prolonged period of time. Alcoholics are not the best judges of what emotions they are feeling at any given time. Someone who simply may have forgotten to eat and has been suffering from insomnia, may become fearful and anxious over something that otherwise wouldn't be given a second thought.

- **Hungry** - Don't get too hungry. For a reason we cannot explain, there seems to be in the alcoholic a peculiar psycho physiological relationship between hunger and the urge to drink. On some occasions, we would eat a big dinner and then find that it literally destroyed our desire to drink afterwards. Conversely, and eventually more often, we avoided eating because we knew it would interfere with our drinking. And so, when you are hungry, eat. Simple and important.

- **Angry** - Don't get too Angry. Wow! Of all things to tell an alcoholic! But we don't have to be in the program very long to realize that anger, righteous or not, is better left to those who can handle it. Borrowing from Father John Doe: "Let the other guy get mad. If somebody calls me a SOB, either I am or I ain't. If I am, So What? If I ain't, why should I make myself one by getting mad about it?" We can't afford to get angry - especially at other people.

- **Lonely** - Don't get too Lonely. Members of the psychiatric profession tend to equate loneliness with boredom, and I am inclined to agree. If there is any one thing that must be included in the alcoholic's life before he can once again become whole, it is worthwhile activity. This may be helping others, his career, or anything else. But such activity must be present in order to fulfill his existence and eliminate loneliness. Under any conditions, Loneliness is the mother of self-pity and the ultimate end is resentment and drinking. The rule of Thumb? Do something!

- **Tired** - Don't get too Tired. In its effect, the last ingredient or direction in this rule is not too different from the first. Physical fatigue will affect both our bodies and our minds adversely and will thereby lower our defenses against the urge to drink if there is any possibility at all of such a desire being present, consciously or subconsciously. And there the rule of thumb is "When you are tired, put the body down!" (Remember that slogan: "Easy Does It"?)

When we confuse or ignore basic needs, we may be complicating what is really a simple issue. Remember, the H.A.L.T. needs are simple, basic needs. Take a look at these first and see if they need to be addressed. This goes along the lines of "Keep is Simple". This is a great portable and practical tool for self-care and recovery.

Better keep yourself clean and bright; you are the window through which you must see the world. -George Bernard Shaw

Hungry
Angry
Lonely
Tired

Sober Living Alternatives

The ultimate lesson all of us have to learn is unconditional love, which includes not only others but ourselves as well. -Elizabeth Kubler-Ross

Everyday life in early sobriety can be tough, even for the most dedicated and willing of the bunch. Add to that, having to deal with the mountain of problems that many of us walk in with, and it's no wonder that sometimes an extra level of support isn't welcome. Sober Living Alternatives, such as halfway houses, 3/4 houses and just "sober houses" fit this bill nicely. They actually can fill quite a few needs and should be considered if:

- You are leaving treatment and have no direction and no place to live
- You did not go to treatment but would like a safe, clean, sober environment to live in while starting recovery in a 12 Step program
- Your home environment is not conducive to recovery (ie - people drink, aren't supportive, etc)

So, just what is a Sober Living home? Well, they're not treatment centers. You will pay to live there, although the cost varies and some are extremely affordable. What they do is to provide a clean and sober environment for the recovering alcoholic whose environment can play a significant role in whether or not he drinks or uses again. A sober living home puts the individual in an atmosphere away from old friends and stomping grounds that may act as triggers and places him in a new environment with a new support system. Generally, the length of stay at a sober living house is three to six months, with admission and discharge typically being voluntary decisions.

There are several different types of sober living environments that you can investigate. Most sober living homes are same-sex, either all-male or all-female but I do know of a few that are co-ed. There are also what are called Halfway Houses and 3/4 Houses. The difference between these is generally in the strictness of the rules. Halfway

Kickstart Your Recovery

Houses are going to have stricter rules and more accountability, although both certainly have plenty of each. There may be a tighter curfew in a halfway house and more frequent drug testing. What all sober living facilities have in common are these elements:

- Residents live in the home and follow very clear house rules
- They generally all promote 12-Step Programs and require attendance at meetings
- There is a House Manager, and sometimes staff, that implements the structure and provides supervision
- Provides a secure, safe structure intended for the long-term recovery of residents
- Is a Communal Living environment where you will likely share a room with another resident and share in household duties such as cooking and cleaning
- Requires Accountability by meeting clear obligations (often spelled out in a Contract), such as house duties, meeting attendance, maintaining employment, paying bills, and staying sober.
- Zero Tolerance policy for breaking rules.

Sober living facilities have gained immense popularity these days for they offer amenities in a cost-effective way. The "community living" methods followed here enable the residents to share space with each other. The different responsibilities which they are required to carry out help them regain their self-esteem and increase their sense of accountability. All of this serves in diverting their attention to positive things during the phase when relapse remains a matter of serious concern. If you think that one of these facilities could be of benefit in kickstarting your recovery, definitely check them out.

Don't use your past as an excuse to miss out on your future. -Alan Cohen

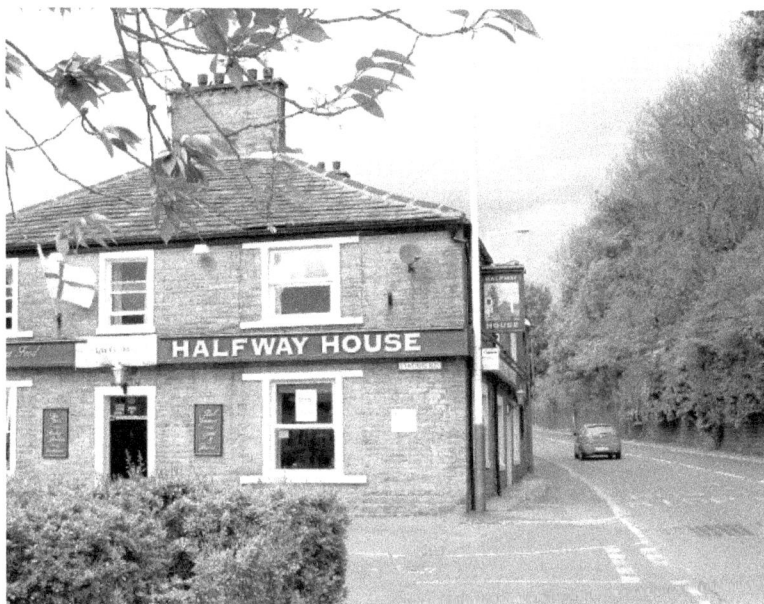

Learning to Have Fun Again

People rarely succeed unless they have fun in what they are doing. Dale Carnegie

I seriously wonder how many people actually just jump straight to this section of the book and forget about everything else. This was a major concern of mine. Despite the fact that I hadn't been happy or had any sort of "fun" in years, I was genuinely concerned that getting sober was going to suck all of the fun out of my life for good. Makes sense, right? Uh, hmmmm. Anyway, when people get sober, one of the biggest fears is exactly this. Can I ever have fun again? Will life just be boring as hell? Why do we think this? Well, I know for me that I started getting messed up at such a young age that I forgot how to have fun sober. When you've only really skied, vacationed, watched sports or gone dancing drunk, it can seem an impossibility to imagine doing those things any other way. Another reason is that we tend to surround ourselves with people that condone this behavior and emulate it, so my drinking and using friends were my only point of reference. I didn't have friends, or at least not ones that I really hung out with, that did these sorts of things sober. All of this being said, learning to have fun sober is a must.

Winning is only half of it. Having fun is the other half. ~ Bum Phillips

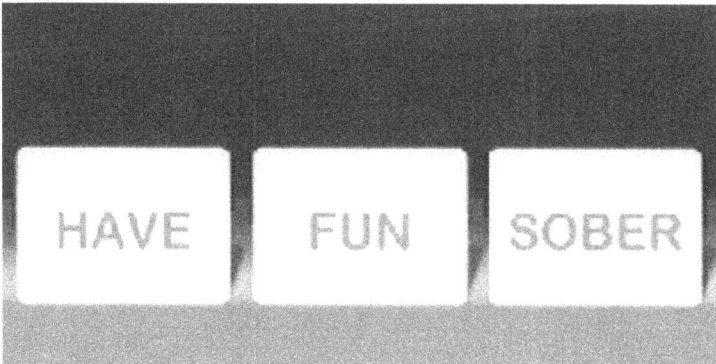

Taite Adams

We Are Not a Glum Lot

. . . we aren't a glum lot. If newcomers could see no joy or fun in our existence, they wouldn't want it. We absolutely insist on enjoying life. We try not to indulge in cynicism over the state of the nations, nor do we carry the world's troubles on our shoulders ALCOHOLICS ANONYMOUS, p. 132

One thing you may have noticed when walking into your first AA meeting was ...laughter. People in AA, and in recovery, have fun. It may be annoying as hell at first, inconceivable, and just downright freaky. The fact is, nearly all of us felt this way when first getting sober. No one enters recovery on a high note, but we quickly discover the things we can't control, the things we can, and most of us find some peace that allows us to relax and enjoy a moment. That moment may turn into a minute and, the next thing you know, you've enjoyed yourself for an entire hour - sober!

The prospect of going from a party animal to sitting at home alone in the corner knitting a sweater doesn't appeal to very many of us. Luckily, this doesn't have to be your reality. Living a sober life probably will no longer involve late night high speed chases with the cops and back alley shady deals but I was pretty grateful to be done with that crap. The definition of "fun" changes with recovery and joy becomes much more enriching and rewarding. The truth is, that if you get sober and don't make the effort to learn how to relax and have fun, it can take serious effort at first, the prospects for long-term sobriety may be limited. Having fun and enjoying life are critical components of recovery.

So, what are some of the "fun" things you can do in sobriety? Actually, the list is pretty endless. I can tell you that people in AA are big on conventions, dances, picnics, pot lucks, camping and (this is huge) EATING. We love to go out to eat. Some of your biggest opportunities to get to know people outside of meetings are by going out to breakfast, lunch or dinner before or after a meeting. This can, easily, become a habit where you will form some solid friendships and then begin doing other things with these people in between meetings.

Kickstart Your Recovery

I have lived in several places in recovery and this is always how it has worked for me. Other things you can do are: go to concerts, go on road trips, exercise, and learn a new skill. Invite people in the fellowship to do these things with you and you will form lifelong bonds and strengthen your support network. Better yet, you'll have a blast!

Why are addicts and alcoholics afraid to let go and have fun? We had to ingest serious amounts of drugs or alcohol to let go of our fears and insecurities. Working the Twelve Steps helps to reduce the fear, allowing us to create bonds in the fellowship with others in recovery, which can also help teach us what the "new fun" looks like. The beauty of recovery is that, if you reach out enough, you will find others who have the same interests as you, and often even the same sense of humor. But first it takes reaching out. This isn't always easy and the people in the meetings are very sympathetic to this. It takes very little effort to get involved. I am painfully shy and have never had a problem getting into the middle of things when I put forth just the tiniest bit of effort. It has always paid off in spades - in laughter, love and new sober experiences.

The average person living to age 70 has 613, 000 hours of life. This is too long a period not to have fun.

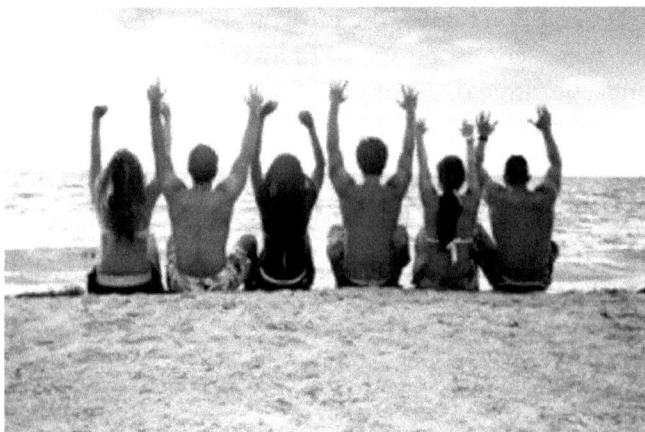

Rule 62 - Seriously, Laugh a Little

I realize that humor isn't for everyone. It's only for people who want to have fun, enjoy life, and feel alive.   -Anne Wilson Schaef

If you hang around AA, you will hear "Rule 62" mentioned occasionally and this particular rule means "Do not take yourself too damn seriously".   Since you won't find it in the literature, here are its origins: Rule 62 was created by a founding member of AA who scoffed at the idea of an Alcoholics Anonymous with "Rules". When a rules committee was formed to discuss a huge list of rules the founding members had come up with (61 to be exact), this man suggested that no rules were necessary for AA, because Alcoholics never follow rules anyway! After much discussion, he suggested that there may be just one rule AAs should follow; and that would be Rule 62, which states: "Do not take yourself too damn seriously!" The committee abandoned the idea of an AA with rules, and today this is the only one that remains - but it is not really a rule, because alcoholics don't like "Rules"!

One thing you will notice if you go to enough meetings and pay attention to what's shared is that people have a tendency to joke sometimes when sharing, to share some very personal details of their pasts in a lighthearted manner and to be a bit self-deprecating in nature. This is not meant to be crass or even egotistical. What has happened is that there has been a shift in perspective in the recovering alcoholic wherein they find that their experiences are no longer as shameful as they once thought; their actions were due to the insidious nature of the disease and the realization comes that sharing these things is helpful in their recovery. By not taking themselves so seriously, learning to laugh at their mistakes and being open, a recovering alcoholic is able to let go of a lot of fear and shame and is also able to help others by sharing their experience, strength and hope with others.

The phenomenon of laughter and humor received a lot of attention in 1979 when Norman Cousins published his book *The Anatomy of an Illness* in which he talks about the body's ability to recover from illness and how it is related to the mental attitudes of the person. Laughter was further examined in 2001 when Robert Provine, PhD, wrote his book *Laughter*: A Scientific Investigation. In the book *Provine* examines the multiple sources of laughter, gender differences, and the physiological process that take place when laughter occurs. The author concludes that laughter may indeed have some therapeutic properties and should be studied further. Laughter is a self soothing, mood altering experience and brings forth joy, happiness, delight and bliss. Laughter is also a physical experience where an individuals blood pressure and heart rate comes down and endorphins, the brains natural painkillers, are released.

The results of many scientific studies on the effects of laughter have led most experts to agree that laughter can provide recovering addicts and alcoholics with an effective tool to begin recovering joy in their lives. The addicts brain is wired to ensure the repetition of activities associated with pleasure or reward. It ultimately seeks the release of dopamine, endorphins and serotonin - known as the happy chemicals. The effect of such a powerful reward strongly motivates people to pursue those substances again and again. Laughter works much the same way. Laughter releases happy chemicals. The mere act of smiling causes the brain to release dopamine, which in turn makes us feel good. And laughter is free! In order to stay sober alcoholics and addicts have to change just one thing - everything! What else could be better than to laugh our way through that!

."*Outsiders are sometimes shocked when we burst into merriment over a seemingly tragic experience out of the past. But why shouldn't we laugh? We have recovered, and have been given the power to help others.*" -Alcoholics Anonymous

You grow up the day you have the first real laugh --at yourself. -Ethel Barrymore

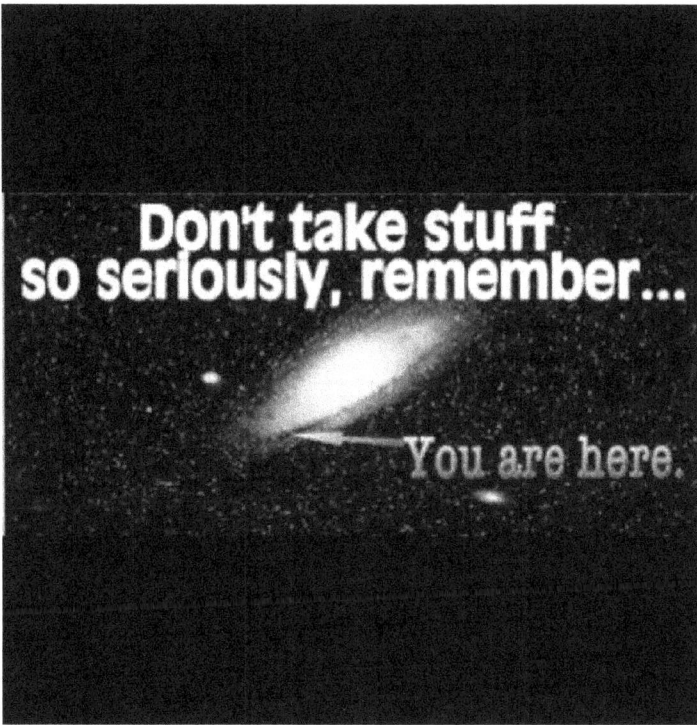

Don't take stuff so seriously, remember... You are here.

Taite Adams

Sober Travel and Vacations

Life is either a daring adventure or nothing. *-Helen Keller*

Many of us dream of once again being able to go on vacations or, better yet, having the ability to take those trips that we only talked about while sitting on the barstool but were too bogged down with our addictions to take. Well, fear not - the sober travel business is HUGE. Choices abound as to what you can do with yourself stone cold sober these days and the sky is the limit.   You can do whatever comes to the imagination, but there are things organized as diverse as sober music festivals, camping, yoga retreats and cruises, vacation rentals and resorts and much more.

Organized sober travel will generally happen through a sober travel agent (there are tons), who can research AA meetings in the location, be sure that tour operators are aware that participants are in recovery, and set up sober activities. Some sober travel agencies will allow for payment plans so that you can plan your trips with sober groups well in advance and do things such as go on ski trips, golfing, rafting, cruises and even Club Med vacations.

Aside from the organized sober travel groups, most major cruise lines will have "Friends of Bill" meetings on board for anyone who wants to attend.   There are also regional conventions and the International Convention of Alcoholics Anonymous that you can plan to attend. The next International Convention will be in Atlanta in the summer of 2015 (I'll be there).   These are huge celebrations, with over 59,000 people attending the last one in San Antonio.   These only occur once every 5 years but there are states conventions, local conventions and "round-ups" happening constantly. Depending on where you live, you could literally stay busy with these just about every weekend of the year.

I have always loved to travel but many of my trips were a blur or ended up being insanely expensive because of the alcohol bill at the end. Getting to travel and see new places, and re-experience old places, sober has been a blessing. I went on a Sober Cruise after just a few years sober and it was a lot of fun. I met a lot of new people from all over the country. We had meetings on the ship, ate together, went on excursions together and stayed in touch after the trip. I've also travelled around the world, both with companions and alone, in sobriety and have enjoyed myself immensely. It takes a lot of pressure off of the itinerary when you are not worried about hunting down that next drink or drug and can just relax and enjoy the ride. This is one of the biggest benefits of sobriety to me.

"Enjoy life today, it is not a dress rehearsal."

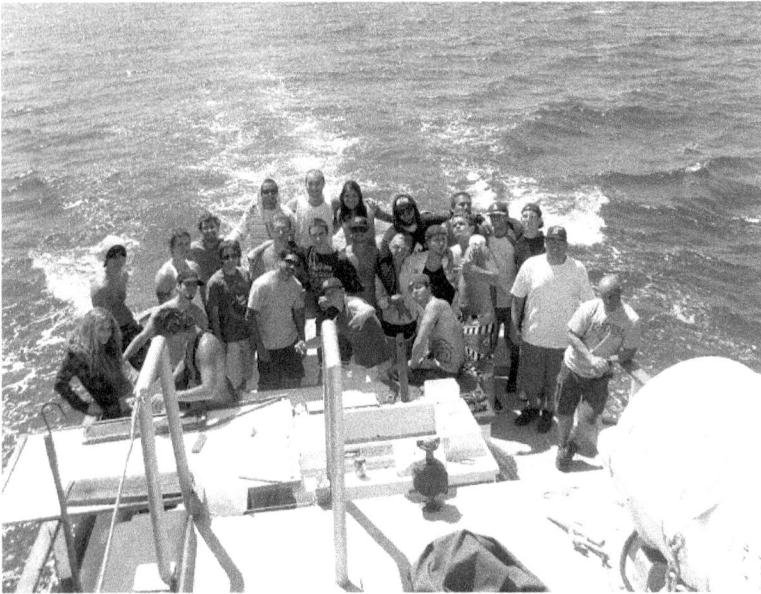

Other Issues

It would be a product of false pride to claim that A. A. is a cure-all, even for alcoholism AS BILL SEES IT, p. 285

There is a lot of confusion and debate in recovery when it comes to "outside" issues and whether or not it is ok to ask for and pursue outside help - and other things like medication. This is an attempt to clarify some of that and, hopefully, not confuse you further. I honestly can't picture anyone, myself included, who walked into AA or a treatment center with the only "problem" being that they had drank too much. There are always underlying causes and conditions that got us to a particular point in time (hopefully a "bottom") and some of us used many different things to excess - alcohol, drugs, food, people. Others of us may have additional psychiatric diagnoses that contributed to our disease and may also play a role in our recovery process. All of these are valid things to take a good hard look at and, if you go to a treatment center, they will certainly help you with this. However, if you do not, you may be left even more lost and confused as to what to about these "other issues" as you move forward. I know I was.

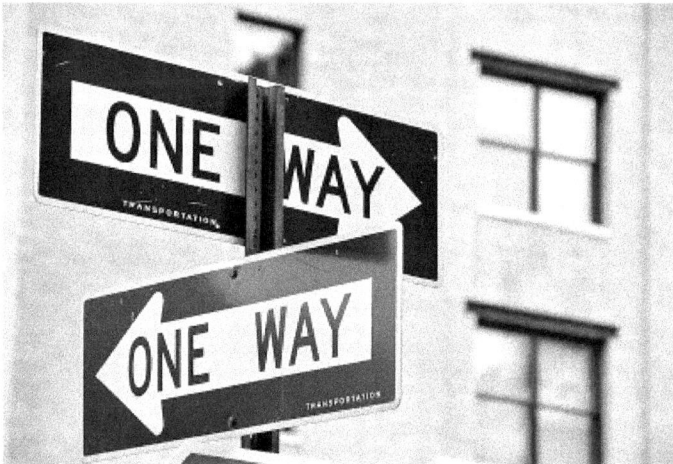

Taite Adams

If it Looks Like a Duck (Other Addictions, Compulsions, etc)

"It's not the load that breaks you down; it's the way you carry it." -Lena Horne

When I came into recovery, and AA, I had a serious prescription drug problem. There is no doubt that I was an alcoholic as I drank like a fish for many many years. However, when I discovered "the pills", I loved them and those are what I stuck with and what took me very quickly to an ugly bottom. I was initially confused and tormented myself over where I belonged. Should I go to NA or AA? What is ok and not ok to talk to about? If I go to AA, am I denying that I had a drug problem and setting myself up for failure? What I learned, very early on, was that it just didn't matter where I went. The fact of the matter was that I was "addicted" to anything that I put in my body that changed the way I felt. It didn't matter if it was pills, booze, cocaine, etc. What mattered was that I finally understood that and was able to really internalize it. At that point, I found the fellowship that I was most comfortable in and made it my home.

AA was my choice because I found that members, for the most part, focused on the solution and on living sober. There isn't a lot talk in meetings about actual "drinking" just for this reason. The idea is to learn how to live sober and be happy, not to sit around and tell war stories about the good old days - they weren't good. I was also able to make this mental shift, where every time I said "My name is Taite, I'm an Alcoholic", it was all-encompassing. This, to me, means that I can't put anything in my body that is going to change the way I feel. I do this out of respect for the fellowship that has saved my life and its Traditions.

There is no doubt that there are thousands just like me, members of AA, who can claim to be addicted to many things. Working the 12 Steps of AA doesn't just ensure that I'll live a happy and useful life without wanting to pick up a drink again. It also ensures that I can have an incredible life free of many of these outside compulsions that took over and ruled me from the inside out. Not only do I not have the compulsion to drink, I don't want to do drugs today, lie to family members or friends, or spend money that I don't have. I don't have to go to NA for drugs, CA for cocaine and so on. However, I am free to do so if I want. I do have friends that are in several fellowships and some are helpful for non-substance problems, such as with gambling and sex. This is certainly available to anyone, but not always necessary.

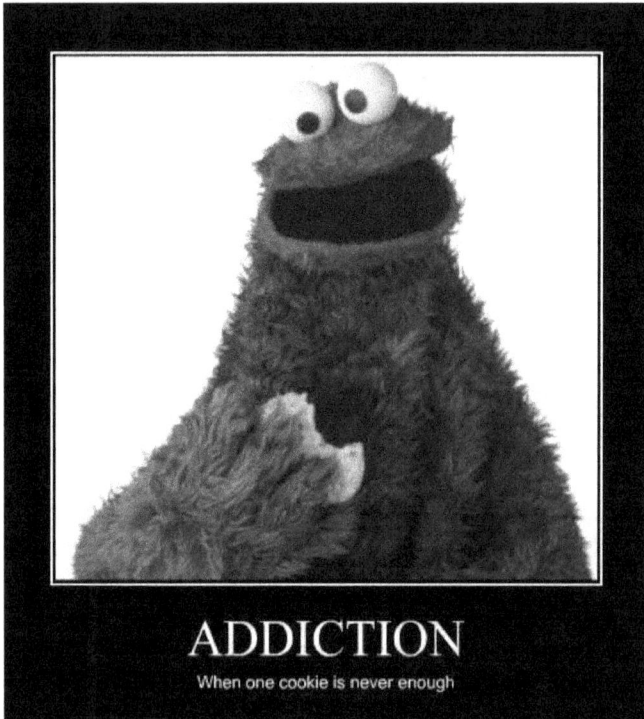

ADDICTION

When one cookie is never enough

Taite Adams

Seeking Outside Help

When you're drowning, you don't say 'I would be incredibly pleased if someone would have the foresight to notice me drowning and come and help me,' you just scream. John Lennon

A separate issue entirely occurs when a newly recovering person has other simultaneous issues that are affecting their recovery. These may be known in advance, may be diagnosed during treatment or in some cases may not come to light until well into sobriety. The fact is that addicts can be pretty complicated folks, and despite AAs success in helping alcoholics get and stay sober, AA alone is not enough to manage the host of complications that an alcoholic may have. That is why AA is very clear about separating itself from medicine and psychiatry, pointedly telling members to get "outside help" when necessary.

Research has proven that people with alcohol or other drug disorders often suffer from a bouquet of descriptive acronyms and psycho jargon that has replaced AAs placid "character defects" mentioned so often in the Big Book - "duel disorders," "comorbid disorders," "MICA" (mentally ill chemical abusers) and substance abusers with "SMI" (serious mental health illness), to name a few. The newest term is "co-occurring disorder." The percentages are a bit daunting as well; about 16% of the US population suffers from substance abuse problems. In people with mental health disorders, the number is almost twice as high: 29%. Forty-seven percent of schizophrenics and 56% of people with bipolar disorders have a substance abuse disorder. Almost 80% of alcoholics experience depression at some time in their lives, and 30% meet the diagnostic requirements for major depression. As many as one-third of people entering treatment for substance abuse issues meet the requirements for Post-Traumatic Stress Syndrome (PTSD).

So how does a member know when it is time to seek "outside help"? Well, if you have been handed one of those nifty diagnoses either before getting sober or in treatment, that would be a good indication that you may want to check in with your doctor and let them know what's up. If you don't have a specialist, just start with a General Practitioner and be honest about your situation and where you are at. A great mental health professional for recovering addicts are LADC's (Licensed Alcohol and Drug Counselor), which many times can either be psychiatrists or medical doctors with additional training in chemical dependency and abuse issues. It's well-known that diagnosing and treating many "co-concurring" disorders can be difficult until the patient has been sober at least 6 months, when you can get a clearer picture of what they are really like.

One of the many dangers of not managing co-occurring disorders, of course, is relapse. Active addiction amplifies the co-occurring disorders so that sobriety must indeed come first if the sufferer is going to have any hope of getting better. But the other side is that untreated depression, anxiety or mania can trigger relapse. The American Association of Marriage and Family Therapists has set up an online service for people in recovery to "seek outside help." The TherapistLocator.net website is designed specifically to put those in need of services in touch with those who provide them. If you feel like you need Outside Help, don't be afraid to get it.

"Asking for help does not mean that we are weak or incompetent. It usually indicates an advanced level of honesty and intelligence." Jim Rohn

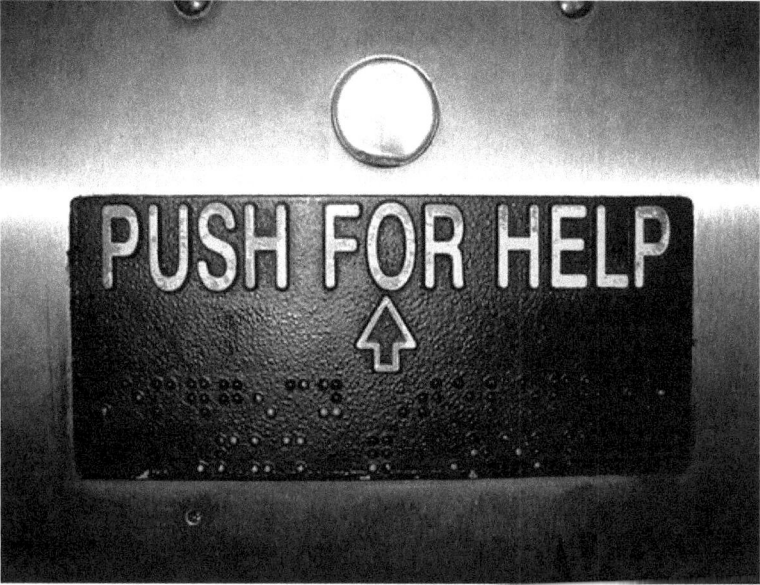

Where Do I Go From Here?

It is good to have an end to journey towards; but it is the journey that matters, in the end. -Ursula K. LeGuin

If not properly schooled in addiction and recovery matters, as I was not for a very long time, many of us may believe that a brief "time out" from life and using is going to be all that is required to set things right again. If you've paid attention to any of the prior chapters in which I've stated more than a few times that, "the only thing you need to change is - everything", there may be a bit of a hint that this just isn't the case. An entire Aftercare industry has been built on this premise and it's been shown, time and again, that recovery from the disease of alcoholism is an ongoing process. Those who feel they have "graduated" or have arrived are in for a rude awakening.

It is easy to let up on the spiritual program of action and rest on our laurels. We are headed for trouble if we do, for alcohol is a subtle foe. ALCOHOLICS ANONYMOUS, p. 85

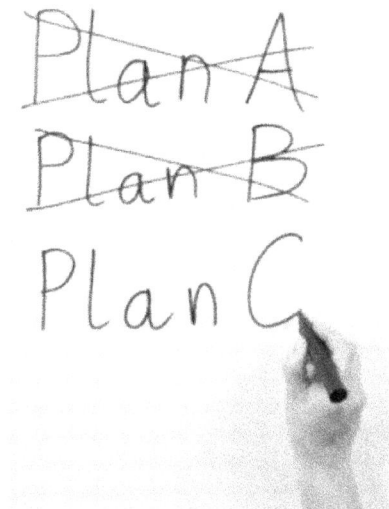

Taite Adams

I Feel Much Better Now - Thanks for the Advice, Phone Numbers, Coffee and 3 Meetings. See Ya

. . . no society of men and women ever had a more urgent need for continuous effectiveness and permanent unity. We alcoholics see that we must work together and hang together, else most of us will finally die alone. ALCOHOLICS ANONYMOUS, p. 562

I heard early on that this disease is "cunning, baffling and powerful". How true that is! Addiction is a disease that continually tells us that we "don't have a disease" and that everything will be just fine, we can handle it or we're better now. I remember one of the first times that I realized that I couldn't stop on my own - that I needed help. I had just gotten a new, high-powered job (God knows how) and wanted to start my life "fresh" with it. I figured that I would check myself into the hospital for a quick 3-4 day Detox, walk out and just start life over again fresh. I set everything up, didn't tell anyone what was going on because "I could handle it", and prepared for my new life.

I left work one afternoon and went straight to the hospital, checked in and slept while detoxing for days. At the end of those 3 days, I felt great and had a new lease on life. When I was supposedly "clean", I put on my business suit to go straight to work, walked out of that hospital and was messed up again before lunch time. I was baffled, ashamed and completely demoralized. What I didn't understand at that time was that the same person that walked into that hospital was going to use again. Not only did I have to change, but I had to keep changing and growing in order to stay sober and live a happy life.

It is tempting for those of us that have made it through detox, a treatment center or 90 days in AA to declare that their problems are solved. Many people actually start feeling better quite quickly and problems start to fade away as well. It is also tempting to pat ourselves on the back for finally getting help. It is a great achievement but is not the end in itself by a long shot. While I hate recovery statistics because they can be depressing (and inaccurate), here's one to take note of: Up to 50% of those who make it through an addiction treatment program will later relapse. Those who relapse may never get another opportunity to recover. Again, once we start feeling better, many of us forget that this is a fatal disease.

If you did go to a treatment center, you most certainly would have been prepared for this with relapse prevention counseling and the offering of Aftercare services if they are available. If you didn't go to treatment, that's fine. You can receive all of the help and guidance that you need through the support network that you build in AA and through outside counseling if you feel that you need it. One of the most important things to remember is that recovery is always going to be a process and a journey. There is no final destination.

"People who don't go to meetings never get to see what happens to people who don't go to meetings."

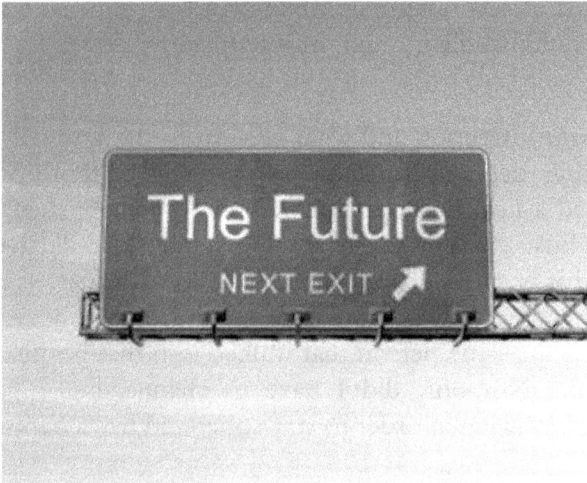

Taite Adams

Do I Have to Do This Forever?

This is not an overnight matter. It should continue for our lifetime.
ALCOHOLICS ANONYMOUS, p. 84

To keep the lamp burning we have to keep putting oil in it. -Mother Teresa

One knock on AA is often the idea of going to meetings "forever"; Some people will ask "Do I have to do this forever?". Well, do what forever? Live without alcohol and drugs ruling your life? Have a happy, rich and fulfilling existence? Have friends that like you, trust you and care about you, that you like, trust and care about?! Build lifelong relationships that are productive and fulfilling? The reason people ask this question is the fear of change and simply not understanding the potential that lies before them.

One thing alcoholics tend to have in common is a need to stay motivated and to avoid boredom. When first getting sober, it's easy to be highly motivated. This new life is exciting and the world appears full of possibilities. As time passes, the newness of recovery can tend to fade. After the first couple of years, addicts have sat through hundreds, if not thousands, of meetings; worked the steps; had commitments; and maybe even picked up a sponsee or two. Many might think they've got the problem all sewn up. Even when sober life is so much more rewarding than the life of an active alcoholic or addict, we can begin to take things for granted. If motivation to stay sober and work a program begins to wane, the risk of relapse increases. This is particularly true if we make the mistake of slipping back into a pattern of trying to do it on our own, without support.

Long term sobriety is the gold standard of success in beating alcoholism. There are plenty of people who drift in and out of recovery, only getting a small taste of a better life before slipping back into the grip of addiction. For the newcomer, the big question in early recovery becomes: "How can I make this last?" or "How can I turn recovery into a lifestyle?" These questions all point toward the same goal of achieving long term, meaningful sobriety. A few common factors that I've seen in those that have been able to achieve this long term sobriety are these:

- **Strength of Commitment** - Simply dabbling in recovery isn't going to cut it. Those who stick around generally talk about how heavily they were involved in AA in their early years of sobriety. This level of commitment can been viewed as an outward reflection of what is driving you on the inside towards of life of sobriety.

- **Willing to Follow Direction** - Recovery is simply following a set of directions, or suggestions, to help you live a sober life. Those who have been successful in achieving long term sobriety tend to emphasize their strong willingness to follow whatever direction was given to them, whether it made sense or not. This also speaks to a profound level of desperation that is necessary to surrender and begin this journey.

- **One Day at a Time Philosophy** - People in recovery know that they never have to drink or use again ...Just for today. It is helpful to know that if we can just make it through today without drinking, then tomorrow will provide us with a fresh start and things will likely take care of themselves. Many in recovery have learned the power of living in the moment, or the present and a popular book on this subject is Eckhart Tolle's "The Power of Now".

- **Spiritual Experience** - This is very important and what the program (12 Steps) of recovery aims to lead you to. Behavioral approaches and cognitive therapies work great for treating "problem drinkers" or "drug abusers," but for real alcoholics and drug addicts, a complete psychic change in personality is necessary to overcome their problem. This is not the same as religious conversion. The vital spiritual experience is characterized, among other things, by overcoming self-centeredness, and is maintained by working with others in recovery.

- **Balance** - Addicts and alcoholics are experts at unbalancing their lives. While we may get sober, we may become workaholics, shopaholics, exercise fanatics or video game addicts. What we do not know how to do is find true balance and recovery offers us tools to do this, giving us the desire to live a "normal" balanced, healthy life. Many with long-term sobriety have made great strides in this area.

If motivation is an issue for you already, consider the above factors and see how they are being applied in your recovery right now, if at all. Also, take a look at your expectations. Some individuals have expectations of recovery that are too low. This means that they are prepared to settle for less than what is actually possible. It is important that people have goals in their sobriety and that they work towards achieving these. I heard in the beginning, and continue to hear, that if you set down your goals for yourself in sobriety about what you thought was possible, you would sell yourself short by a mile. This is very true in my experience and in so many others that I have had the joy of observing over the years.

"From experience, I've realized that I cannot go back and make a brand-new start. But through A.A., I can start from now and make a brand-new end.'
— Alcoholics Anonymous

I'M GONNA MAKE
THE REST OF MY LIFE,
THE BEST OF MY LIFE.

Taite Adams

The Miracle Mother Load

"To this day, I am amazed at how many of my problems - most of which had nothing to do with drinking, I believed - have become manageable or have simply disappeared since I quit drinking." — *Alcoholics Anonymous*

It is astonishing in this world how things don't turn out at all the way you expect them to! -Agatha Christie

At the end of my drinking and using, I honestly just thought that it would be a miracle if I would be able to go one day without the stuff. That seemed inconceivable to me at the time as I had been living in pure survival mode for so long. Go to enough meetings and you are bound to hear "Don't quit 5 minutes before the miracle happens". If you are having one of those days, these platitudes can be so irritating. However, I had left such a pile of shit in my wake when I came into recovery, that I would have been happy with a semi-miracle or 1/4-miracle at that point. I just nodded my head and kept trudging on. The things that I heard and soon experienced astounded me.

Miracles are instantaneous, they cannot be summoned, but come of themselves, usually at unlikely moments and to those who least expect them. -Katherine Anne Porter

I am realistic –
I expect
miracles.

Dr. Wayne Dyer

Taite Adams

Miracles Happen

"When I stopped living in the problem and began living in the answer, the problem went   away."
— *Alcoholics Anonymous*

When most people think of the word "miracle", they think of something that is a welcome event that is possibly divinely inspired, or an event that defies the laws of nature.   Whether or not some of the things that we see happen in the lives of people that come into recovery fit nicely into this little box or not, they certainly feel miraculous when they occur in our lives and you'd be hard pressed to argue the case against someone who has experienced them.   In fact, the most touching and amazing miracles are those that have to do with people gaining the ability to truly love and serve others, and how their lives take on new meaning.   To see the metamorphosis of some pretty broken people into strong, compassionate and hopeful human beings is a gift in itself.

While this all may sound very touchy feely to the newcomer, it's nothing to shake a stick at.   On a more physical plane, however, miracles happen on a daily basis for people who get sober and continue to do the right thing.   I am living proof and I see it happen for others constantly.   Very serious illnesses resolve themselves, job situations are fixed and family conflicts are mended.   Remember, I wasn't on any sort of winning streak when I got sober.   I had no job, no place to live, was losing my child and was facing prison time.   It was a series of miracles, in my eyes, that I was able to find a place to live and a job right out of treatment, I was able to keep my 3 year old child in my life and I did not end up spending another day in jail.   I see these same things (call them whatever you want) happen in the lives of others all the time.   The fact of the matter is that rewarding things happen for people who, finally, put their recovery first.

These miracles in sobriety are just the tip of the iceberg.   Recovery teaches us that living in appreciation, forgiveness and compassion are interrelated.   Once you learn to forgive yourself and others, releasing all the shame you have been carrying, finding your purpose will be much easier. You will have opened up a space in your heart for true compassion which can only lead to a profound appreciation for your sobriety. When your heart is open, anything and everything is possible. I have seen many people release their resentments towards people, places, and things; letting them go allowing for positive changes to occur.

Finally, learning to let go of resistance and attachments is about not being glued to having things turn out exactly as you envisioned them to be. It is about being open and willing to whatever comes your way so that you do not live in perpetual disappointment when things don't go as you so eloquently planned. Once I became open to wherever my life (career, relationships, etc) was going to take me, more opportunities came forth. By continuing on this journey and remaining open, we continue to allow these miracles to be created in all areas of our lives.

Such is the paradox of A.A. regeneration: strength arising out of complete defeat and weakness, the loss of one's old life as a condition for finding a new one. A.A. COMES OF AGE, p. 46

THE MOST **INCREDIBLE** THING ABOUT **MIRACLES** IS THAT **THEY HAPPEN.**

G.K. CHESTERTON

Giving It Away

. . . he has struck something better than gold. . . . He may not see at once that he has barely scratched a limitless lode which will pay dividends only if he mines it for the rest of his life and insists on giving away the entire product. ALCOHOLICS ANONYMOUS, p. 129

Make yourself a blessing to someone. Your kind smile or pat on the back just might pull someone back from the edge. -Carmelita Elliott

If you are new to this, the prospect of jumping in and helping others or giving away something that you haven't yet "gotten" may seem precarious. No worries, you'll get there. But if you jump back to the chapter that talks about "**What is AA?**", you'll remember that the entire organization was built on the premise of one alcoholic helping another. By our very nature, we are defiant and mistrusting of anyone in authority telling us just what to do, how to live, how to act, what to say or how to think. What works is hearing the actual experience, strength and hope of someone who has the same malady and has walked the same path before us. I would venture to guess that you probably would not have purchased (or downloaded) this book were it not written by someone who has "been there". Likewise, the personal experiences that I have related throughout the book have likely helped a few people at least to relate to the material a little bit better. That is how this works.

Regardless, recovering people who dedicate their time to helping others are not doing this for purely self-less reasons. Instead they have come to realize that by helping others they can help themselves as well. Though there is plenty of debate about what works and what doesn't with regards to recovery, there is little disputing that helping others who have drug or alcohol addiction problems can be very helpful to one's own recovery. There is a saying that many in recovery circles repeat that goes, "When I got busy, I got better." What it means is, in their effort to maintain sobriety, they found that doing service work to help others actually helped them stay clean and sober. Now there is some scientific research that backs up the notion that helping others helps alcoholics and addicts become and stay sober.

Maria E. Pagano, PhD, of Case Western Reserve University School of Medicine, in a published review cited several empirical studies that support the "helper therapy principle", or the idea that when someone helps another person with a similar condition, they help themselves. Dr. Pagano and colleagues evaluated the decade long of treatment outcomes using data from a single site in Project MATCH, the largest multi-site randomized clinical trial on behavioral treatments of alcoholism sponsored by the National Institute on Alcohol Abuse and Alcoholism. Results showed that participation in Alcoholics Anonymous-related Helping (AAH) produced lowered alcohol use and increased interest in others at each subsequent follow-up assessment. "The AAH findings suggest the importance of getting active in service, which can be in a committed 2-month AA service position or as simple as sharing one's personal experience in recovery to another fellow sufferer." This study also found that alcoholics engaged in AAH did more step-work and attended more meetings than those not helping others. In effect, AAH strengthens the commitment to the program that many newcomers have difficulty with in the beginning.

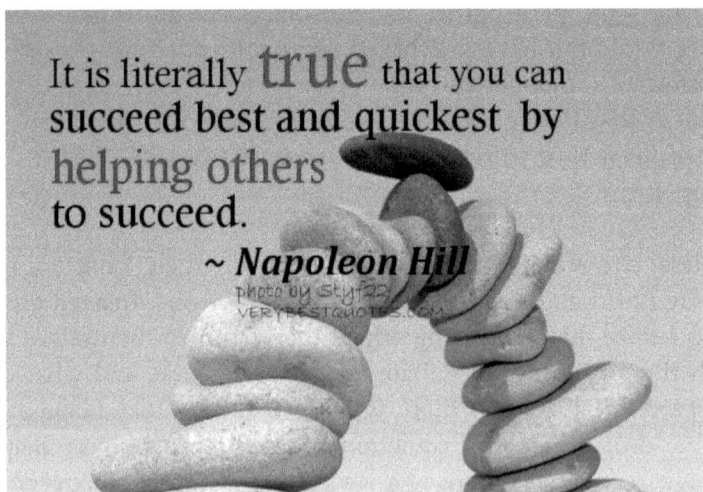

It is literally *true* that you can succeed best and quickest by helping others to succeed.
~ *Napoleon Hill*

Not sure where to start? Many of us aren't so you're certainly not alone. Simple answer, just ask. However, as further explanation Alcoholics Anonymous is a non-profit organization. It relies completely on the service of its members. Each group is an autonomous unit and it is up to the members to ensure that everything runs smoothly. These groups could not survive if members were not prepared to take on unpaid responsibilities. Newly sober people may be asked to make the coffee or tea, or welcome other newcomers. Those who are sober longer may be given responsibilities such as acting as the meeting secretary or treasurer. Members will also often take turns as the main speaker at the meeting or acting as chairperson. Some individuals will take on additional responsibilities such as telephone service or sponsorship.

Helping other people in recovery is one of the most effective ways to stay motivated. In Alcoholics Anonymous, they say that you have to give it away to keep it, and this is what helping others is about. It reminds people in recovery about where they have come from, and what they would be going back to if they ever relapsed. Also, alcoholics have a tendency to be very self-absorbed. By thinking about and helping others, this allows them to take the focus off of themselves and get a change in perspective. Helping others also helps to continue to build self-esteem as the giver feels that they are giving something back to society. Of key importance here, however, is that by helping other people stay sober, the individual continues to strengthen their own recovery.

The only ones among you who will be really happy are those who will have sought and found how to serve. -Albert Schweitzer

Try to be a rainbow
in someone's cloud.

~ Maya Angelou

Afterword

While getting sober in itself was a miracle in my book, the life that I have been given as a result is second to none. If someone were to tell me (someone very well may have) that I would be able to live in such a beautiful place, have such lovely people in my life and not think about drinking and drugging all the time, I would have thought that they were trying to sell me a load of goods. It really is so hard to imagine that things can get better, much less really really good, when caught under the mire of addiction.

I can tell you that I will be forever grateful for that moment of clarity that I finally had, the one in which I was able to put down the shovel and stop digging the hole that I was standing in. From that moment on, I never had to be alone again and everything took on a whole new light. It took losing everything that I lost to get to that point and that's ok. I can appreciate that and it gives me lots of material to share with others and hopefully give something back. This book was as much a healing and clarifying exercise for me as it was just another avenue to relay my experiences and hopefully help someone who is still suffering. They say we reach our "bottom" when what we just lost or are about to lose is more important than that next drink or drug. This was certainly the case for me. My hope is that this is enough for you as well.

The following pages contain some resources and links that I have put together for your use. Best of luck as you continue to your journey, wherever it may take you.

-Taite A.

Recovery Resources

Treatment Centers

There are no "public" websites that offer treatment center, detox and sober living directories. Unfortunately, any site you find will be filled with "sponsored results". This means rehabs that have paid for ad space. That's not always a bad thing, just not an unbiased thing. The best site I've found is Sober.com. You'll get the sponsored results in your search but you will also get all of the public listings as well, including the government-funded (some free) facilities.

Support Groups

Alcoholics Anonymous (http://aa.org/)
Al-Anon Websites (http://www.al-anon.alateen.org/)
Narcotics Anonymous (http://www.na.org/)
Cocaine Anonymous (http://ca.org/)
Adult Children of Alcoholics (http://www.adultchildren.org/)
Co-Dependence Anonymous (CoDA) (http://www.coda.org/)

Mental Health

National Institute of Mental Health (http://www.nimh.nih.gov/)
Results of biomedical research on mind and behavior.

National Alliance for the Mentally Ill (http://www.nami.org/)
Support for consumers with mental illness

Substance Abuse & Mental Health Services Administration (http://www.samhsa.gov/)

United States Department of Health & Human Services

Government Resources

Single-State Agency (SSA) Directory:
(http://www.recoverymonth.gov/Recovery-Month-
Kit/Resources/Single-State-Agency-SSA-Directory.aspx)
Prevention and Treatment of Substance Use and Mental Disorders – A list of State offices that can provide local information and guidance about substance use and mental disorders, treatment, and recovery in your community.

AMVETS (http://www.amvets.org/)
This organization provides support for veterans and the active military in procuring their earned entitlements. It also offers community services that enhance the quality of life for this Nation's citizens.

Professionals

Intervention Project for Nurses (http://www.ipnfl.org/)
Help for professionals with chemical dependencies.

International Lawyers in Alcoholics Anonymous (ILAA)
(http://www.ilaa.org/)
This organization serves as a clearinghouse for support groups for lawyers who are recovering from alcohol or other chemical dependencies.

International Pharmacists Anonymous (IPA)
(http://home.comcast.net/~mitchfields/ipa/ipapage.htm)
This is a 12-step fellowship of pharmacists and pharmacy students recovering from any addiction.

Taite Adams

Other

AlcoholScreening.org - Website offering an online screening tool to assess drinking patterns. The website offers visitors free confidential online screenings to assess their drinking patterns, giving them personalized feedback and showing them if their alcohol consumption is likely to be within safe limits. AlcoholScreening.org was developed by Join Together, a project of the Boston University School of Public Health, and was launched in April 2001. The website also provides answers to frequently asked questions about alcohol and health consequences, and provides links to support resources and a database of local treatment programs. Disclaimer: This site does not provide a diagnosis of alcohol abuse, alcohol dependence or any other medical condition. The information provided here cannot substitute for a full evaluation by a health professional, and should only be used as a guide to understanding your alcohol use and the potential health issues involved with it.

This Center for Substance Abuse Prevention widget includes a variety of updates on activities relating to underage drinking which is updated regularly with local, state, and national articles published by online sources. (http://www.samhsa.gov/about/csap.aspx)

NCADD: (http://ncadd.org/) The National Council on Alcoholism and Drug Dependence, Inc. (NCADD) and its Affiliate Network is a voluntary health organization dedicated to fighting the Nation's #1 health problem – alcoholism, drug addiction and the devastating consequences of alcohol and other drugs on individuals, families and communities.

American Council for Drug Education (http://www.acde.org/) Educational programs and services for teens, parents, and educators

About the Author

Taite Adams is a successful marketer and published author who has traded in the high cost of low living for a much more peaceful, and rewarding, life. Free of alcohol and drugs for over a decade and an active member of Alcoholics Anonymous, Taite (not her real name) enjoys living a sober life and sharing those joys with her family, friends and people looking for a better way to live. She is an avid boater, licensed Coast Guard Captain and prolific traveler. While her bucket list remains long, each day brings a shining new opportunity to cross something off the list or discover something new - and for that she remains forever grateful. **Check out our active Facebook Page: Taite Adams Recovery Books.**

Opiate Addiction has reached epidemic proportions in this country and is something that Taite is intimately familiar with. Read her bestselling book, now in its 3rd edition, chronicling this insidious killer and laying the pathway for freedom from its grip.

Should you require additional assistance with your home detox, be sure to pick up Taite's popular book, Safely Detox From Alcohol and Drugs at Home, also on Amazon.com.

If you or a loved one are in recovery from alcoholism or addiction and want to learn more about emotional sobriety, check out Taite's book titled Restart Your Recovery, also on Amazon.com.

It's hard to miss mention in the media of the drug Molly and the controversy surrounding its use and its ingredients. There is plenty of confusion there as well. Check out Taite's latest book, called Who is Molly? for the latest info on this drug and its dangers.

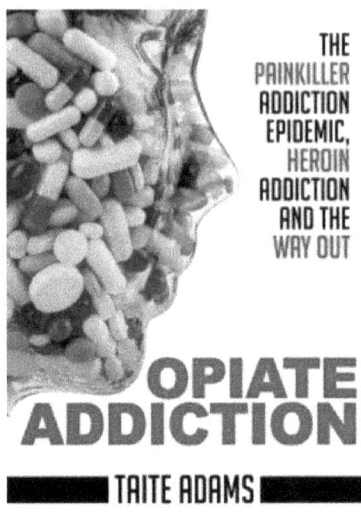

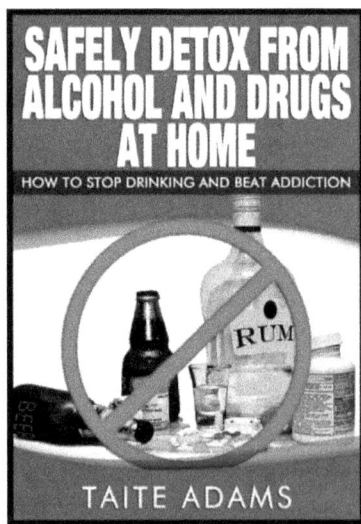

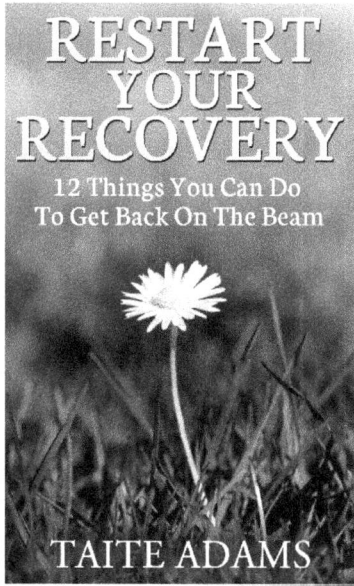

RESTART YOUR RECOVERY
12 Things You Can Do To Get Back On The Beam
TAITE ADAMS

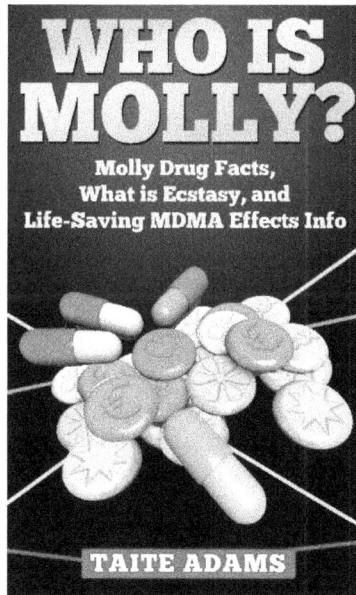

WHO IS MOLLY?
Molly Drug Facts, What is Ecstasy, and Life-Saving MDMA Effects Info
TAITE ADAMS

.....sample of Taite Adams Best Selling book - **Opiate Addiction - The Painkiller Addiction Epidemic, Heroin Addiction and the Way Out**

Preface

The world of opiate addiction is ever-changing and has a lot to do with market conditions. Supply and demand and basic economics play a greater role than many people realize in which drugs come in and out of fashion at a particular point in time. Regardless of which form of opiates are popular at the present moment, there is little doubt that opiates will always be one of the most widely abused classes of drugs. Whether it be Vicodin, Oxys, Perc 30s, methadone or heroin, the opiate addict will generally take what they can get their hands on and then abuse the hell out of it.

Opiates have a very long and rich history of being "in fashion", later shunned by society and then finding their medicinal use for the management of pain. It was this rise in the use of prescription opiate painkillers, however, that has brought about what the CDC is now calling an epidemic of prescription drug addiction. In fact, in 2011 nearly 1.8 million Americans were addicted to some form of prescription painkiller, more than those addicted to cocaine and heroin combined.   I had already been clean from my opiate addiction for over 10 years by this time, yet the memory of the day to day struggle, the terror and hopelessness are still fresh in my mind.   This is not something that I expect to ever forget and it was interesting to re-live some of it and learn a few new "tricks" in the writing of this book.

What scares the hell out of me more than anything else is the rising problem, in epidemic proportions, of heroin use in this country as a direct result of prescription opiate addiction. There is no doubt that prescription painkillers serve as a gateway to heroin use and this is deadly. While abuse of prescription pills for pain was reported to be going down in 2011, according to the national survey on drug use and health, heroin use was reported to be increasing. In fact, in 2011, nearly 200,000 people tried heroin for the first time. In 2014, it's use and abuse is nearly out of control.

If you or a loved one are addicted to opiates, this book is for you. In it you can learn more about the drugs that you have been taking, their effects on your body and mind and what you can do to break free. There is information on opiate maintenance programs as well as warnings on their long-term use and some good information about opiate detox and making treatment center decisions. Recovery from opiate addiction isn't easy but it is absolutely possible and I have found that it is infinitely simpler and more fulfilling than that of the day to day life of a hopeless opiate addict.

The Opiate Addiction Epidemic

Nobody will laugh long who deals much with opium: its pleasures even are of a grave and solemn complexion. -Thomas de Quincey

Most people think that they have a clear picture in their mind of what a drug addict is but generally, when it comes to opiate addiction, what you get couldn't be further from that image. Opiate addicts do not fit a general stereotype as the drug does not discriminate. Because of the nature of opiate addiction, it strikes across age, ethnic and economic groups and then pulls each and every one of those stricken down with equal measure.

The CDC recently reported that opiate addiction is now America's fastest growing drug problem, with the total number of painkillers prescribed in a single year enough to medicate every adult living in the U.S. around the clock. While true that heroin is the most widely used illegal opiate, it's a fact that prescription opiate painkillers are equally dangerous and an insidious problem. The World Health Organization (WHO) estimates that approximately two million people in the United States alone are addicted to prescription opiates.

The problem is also not limited to adults, as first use of opiates seems to be getting younger. The National Institute on Drug Abuse (NIDA) reports that an estimated 52 million people, 20% of those aged 12 and older, have used prescription drugs for nonmedical reasons at least once. Also, about 1 in 12 high school seniors reported nonmedical use of the prescription drug Vicodin the past year. About 1 in 20 high school seniors also reported abusing OxyContin. This isn't limited to the younger crowd either. According to a 2011 study by the Substance Abuse and Mental Health Services Administration (SAMHSA), the rate of current illicit drug use in adults aged 50 to 59 increased to 6.3% in 2011 from 2.7% in 2002 with opiates being among the most commonly abused drugs. The total number of opiate prescriptions dispensed by retail pharmacies in the United States rose from 76 million in 1991 to 210 million in 2010.

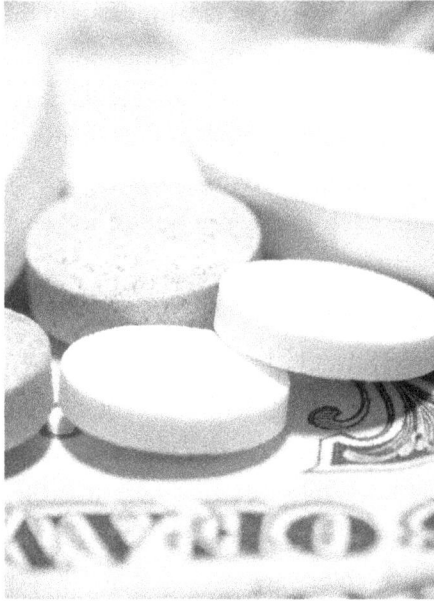

The epidemic of opiate addiction and painkiller addiction has resulted in nearly 16,000 overdose deaths annually. While heroin continues to be a rising problem, opiate addiction in general is not the stereotypical drug problem that many of us think of when we picture the "war on drugs". In fact, many times this involves a patient who began with a legitimate pain issue, an unwitting string of physicians (or not) who are writing these prescriptions, and pharmaceutical companies who are acting within the law. The public consumption of opiates, through legal channels, is costing health insurers over $72 billion annually.

Opiates are a huge problem! ...and growing. Trust me, I know. Most of the time we start taking them for a legitimate pain issue, whether for a root canal or some major surgery. Many times the addiction to them develops over a period of time as a physical dependency develops. With others, however, there is an instantaneous "pull" that these drugs have on you because of the way that they make you feel. They not only take away the physical pain that they were prescribed for, but bring to the table something that you thought you had been looking for for a very long time. This is how it was for me. Those pills became my best friend and my salvation for a time - until they completely owned me.

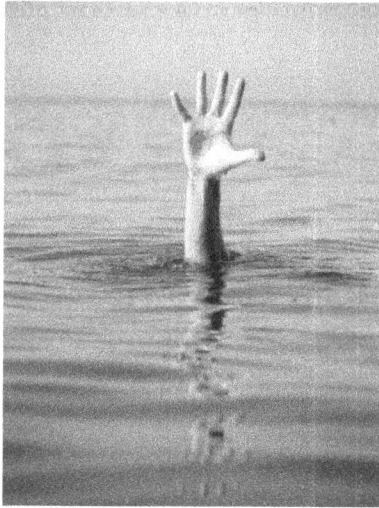

You will find peace not by trying to escape your problems, but by confronting them courageously. You will find peace not in denial, but in victory.   -J. Donald Walters

Kickstart Your Recovery

...keep reading HERE

www.ingramcontent.com/pod-product-compliance
Lightning Source LLC
Chambersburg PA
CBHW060247050426
42448CB00009B/1589

9 780988 987517